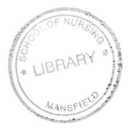

Glossary

AEA: antiendomysial antibody

AGA: antigliadin antibodies

ARA: antireticulin antibodies

DH: dermatitis herpetiformis

EATL: enteropathy-associated T-cell lymphoma

ELISA: enzyme-linked immunosorbent assay

GFD: gluten-free diet

HLA: human leucocyte antigen

IEL: intraepithelial lymphocytes

IL: interleukin

Incidence rate: the number of new cases of a disease occurring in a defined population during a specified period of time

Prevalence: the total number of cases of a disease present in a defined population at a specified time

TNF: tumour necrosis factor

tTG: tissue transglutaminase

Introduction

Advances in medicine are made when astute individuals make observations that have eluded others, or when techniques are developed to investigate hypotheses that previously could not be explored. It is easy to chart the landmarks in our increasing understanding of coeliac disease. In 1888, Samuel Gee put coeliac disease on the map with his paper *On the coeliac affection*. In this delightful account, he described the clinical features in children with remarkable accuracy and predicted with prophetic insight that cure would come from manipulation of the diet. Idiopathic steatorrhoea or non-tropical sprue was much later recognized to be coeliac disease in adults.

The modern era was ushered in when Willem Dicke, a Dutch paediatrician, announced in 1950 that gluten damaged patients with coeliac disease. This led to effective treatment with a gluten-free diet (GFD) and provided researchers with a protein to explore by means of newly emerging techniques in biochemistry and immunology. In the mid-1950s, it was possible for the first time to obtain peroral biopsies of the small intestine, so that coeliac disease could be defined in morphological terms. Abundant fresh tissue became available and was subjected to anatomical, biochemical and immunological scrutiny. At the beginning of the 1970s, genetic markers of coeliac disease were identified. The ability to take intestinal biopsies using fibre-optic endoscopes and the development of serological tests for coeliac disease have greatly facilitated diagnosis in the past two decades.

Coeliac disease is one of the most common lifelong disorders in the western world causing considerable ill health and increased mortality, particularly from malignant complications, the most important of which is lymphoma. Other complications, such as osteoporosis, infertility and neurological disturbances, are increasingly recognized. Careful follow up of patients has drawn attention to the wide spectrum of coeliac disease in terms of clinical manifestations and appearances of the upper small bowel mucosa. These observations have forced changes in the definition and the concept of permanence of the condition. The diagnosis is easily overlooked in those who present, in ever increasing numbers, with non-specific or atypical symptoms. Often the only clue to the diagnosis is the presence of abnormalities revealed by blood tests, such as anaemia, or iron or folate deficiency, or positive results from serological screening tests. For these reasons, a large population of undiagnosed patients exists who are unwell and exposed to various health risks in the community. The challenge for doctors and other healthcare workers is to identify these patients and offer them a GFD that will restore the great majority to full health and may prevent the development of complications. This book offers a concise account of coeliac disease with the hope that it will help to meet this challenge.

CHAPTER 1
Definition

Coeliac disease, or gluten-sensitive enteropathy, is characterized by immune-mediated damage to the jejunal mucosa that is triggered by gluten, a protein in the cereals wheat, rye and barley. Definitions of coeliac disease have revolved around abnormalities found in the jejunal mucosa, and responses to gluten withdrawal and challenge, and the associated clinical reactions. In practice, the diagnosis is usually straightforward and is based on characteristic small bowel biopsy appearance and satisfactory responses to a GFD.

It is clear, however, that the spectrum of gluten sensitivity is wider than previously realized and several forms of coeliac disease are now recognized. Factors, such as the amount of ingested gluten, gastrointestinal infection, or the stress of a pregnancy or operation, may influence the gradual shift from a minimal-change enteropathy to the typical flat lesion characteristic of coeliac disease. Conversely, if the stresses are relieved, the mucosa may return towards normal.

Typical coeliac disease
Typical coeliac disease is a fully expressed gluten-sensitive enteropathy (subtotal villous atrophy), which is found in association with the classical features of malabsorption, such as weight loss, chronic diarrhoea, steatorrhoea and, in infants, failure to thrive.

Atypical coeliac disease
Atypical coeliac disease is a fully expressed gluten-sensitive enteropathy, which is found in association with atypical manifestations. These include lethargy, anaemia, short stature, pubertal delay, arthralgia and infertility.

Silent coeliac disease
Silent coeliac disease is a fully expressed gluten-sensitive enteropathy, which is occasionally found following serological screening in patients who are asymptomatic.

Potential coeliac disease

Potential coeliac disease is a minimal-change enteropathy in which the mucosa has well-formed, normal-looking villi, but subtle abnormalities are present, such as an increased number of intraepithelial lymphocytes (IEL) bearing the γ/δ T cell receptor. Such patients are positive for antiendomysial antibodies (AEA) and can either be well or have intestinal symptoms. In time, they may develop a flat mucosa.

Latent coeliac disease

Latent coeliac disease is the term used to describe patients who have a normal biopsy while on a normal diet, but in whom biopsy findings have revealed a flat or severely damaged mucosa at some time, which recovers on a GFD.

CHAPTER 2
Epidemiology

Coeliac disease is one of the most common, lifelong disorders in western countries. In Europe, the prevalence ranges from 0.3% to 1%, which is higher than for other chronic conditions, such as familial hyper-cholesterolaemia, selective IgA deficiency, type 1 diabetes mellitus and congenital hypothyroidism. Variations in the prevalence of coeliac disease have recently been found in Europe, but are likely to reflect random fluctuations of small-sized samples rather than true differences.

There are not sufficient available data to determine the frequency of coeliac disease outside Europe. In the USA, a country in which coeliac disease has traditionally been considered a rare disorder, the prevalence in blood donors is 0.4%. Similar figures are expected wherever a substantial proportion of the population is of European origin, for example in South America and Australia. For unknown reasons, although it is likely to be linked to genetic factors, coeliac disease appears to be a common disorder in North African (e.g. Algerian and Tunisian) and Middle Eastern populations. In the Saharawis, an Arab population living in the western Sahara, the prevalence of coeliac disease in the general population has recently been found to be as high as 5 or 6%. Coeliac disease is recognized in the Punjab as 'summer diarrhoea', and occurs quite commonly in Asians who reside in Europe. It is unknown among black people.

The coeliac iceberg
Remarkably, only a small proportion of all coeliac patients are diagnosed on clinical grounds (Figure 2.1). Most escape diagnosis unless identified by screening with serological markers, such as antigliadin antibodies (AGA) or the IgA-class AEA.

In a multicentre Italian study, screening with AGA identified seven new biopsy-proven cases of childhood coeliac disease for each known coeliac patient. This also occurs in adult practice. These observations led to the concept of the coeliac iceberg, which is made up of a visible part, representing patients who are clinically diagnosed, usually because they are sick, and a far bigger submerged portion that includes all individuals with

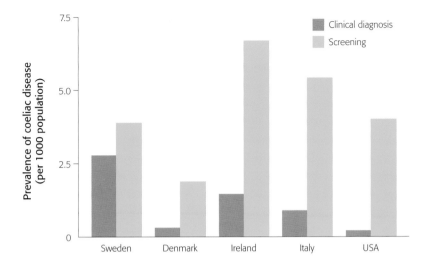

Figure 2.1 In most countries, serological screening has revealed a much higher prevalence of coeliac disease than clinical diagnosis. The only exception is Sweden, where most cases show a typical onset during the first years of life due to the high gluten intake of infants.

gluten-sensitive enteropathy who remain undiagnosed, mostly because of atypical complaints or lack of symptoms altogether (Figure 2.2). It should be noted that the available evidence suggests that all coeliac patients, regardless of the intensity of their symptoms, are exposed to the long-term complications of this condition, such as anaemia, infertility, osteoporosis and lymphoma.

Risk factors

Genetic. The primary role of genetic factors is well established. In identical twins, the concordance for coeliac disease is about 70%, and 5–10% of first-degree relatives are also affected. The major component of the genetic predisposition to coeliac disease resides in the human leucocyte antigen (HLA) region of chromosome 6. Coeliac disease is strongly associated with HLA class II antigens and approximately 90% of cases show a particular DQ2 α/β heterodimer encoded by DQA1*0501 and DQB1*02 alleles inherited in *cis* with DR3 (on the same chromosome) or in *trans* with DR5/DR7 (on different chromosomes). Originally, the DQB1* allele was

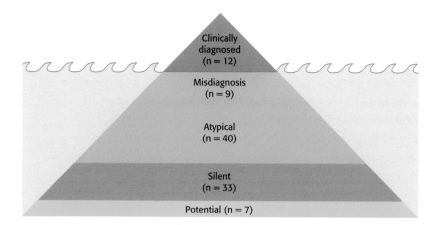

Figure 2.2 The coeliac iceberg in Italy, as revealed by an Italian multicentre study in 1995. Of the 101 individuals with coeliac disease, only 12 had been detected clinically. 'Misdiagnosis' indicates coeliac patients who had resumed a normal diet after a period on a gluten-free diet. Data from Catassi *et al.* 1996.

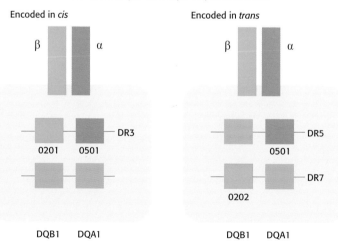

Figure 2.3 Coeliac patients who carry DR3 or DR5/DR7 may express the same HLA-DQ molecule HLA-DQ (α1*0501, β1*02). The genes DQA1*0501 and DQB1*02 may be located in *cis* (on the same chromosome) in DR3 subjects or in *trans* (on different chromosomes) in DR5/DR7 heterozygous individuals.

termed DQB1*0201 but recently it has been found that the DQB1* alleles differ between DR3 and DR7 haplotypes. The former carries DQB1*0201 and the latter DQB1*0202. These differ only at one residue in the membrane proximal domain. This single amino acid substitution at position 135 does not appear to affect function in terms of peptide binding or presentation. The risk alleles are now jointly referred to as DQB1*02 and the β chains as DQβ*02 (Figure 2.3). Most studies to date, however, have reported results in terms of DQB1*0201. The few patients who are DQ2 negative are often HLA-DR4, DR8 positive. The strong linkage disequilibrium between HLA genes, especially between DQ and DR alleles explains the reported association of coeliac disease with the B8, DR3, DR5 and DR7 alleles.

The genetic susceptibility to coeliac disease is only partly explained by HLA alleles. In most European populations, the frequency of DQ2 is high but only a minority of DQ2 positive subjects will develop coeliac disease. Unfortunately, the search for non-HLA genes predisposing to coeliac disease, which may contribute about 60% of the risk, has remained fruitless.

Age. An inverse relationship between the prevalence of coeliac disease and age has been noted in some screening studies. It is not clear whether this reflects a decreased sensitivity of the coeliac disease markers or a 'truly' lower prevalence of this condition in adults.

Gender. The prevalence of coeliac disease is slightly higher in females.

Diet. Coeliac disease only manifests when gluten is present in the diet. In many areas of the world, such as sub-Saharan Africa, East Asia and South America, gluten-containing cereals are not the staple food. Accordingly, coeliac disease will not arise even in genetically susceptible individuals in these areas.

Other risk factors. The prevalence of coeliac disease is increased in patients with a number of conditions:
- type 1 diabetes mellitus (5% of patients are affected)
- other autoimmune disorders, such as liver, thyroid and pulmonary diseases, Sjögren's syndrome and inflammatory bowel disease

- Down's syndrome (4 or 5% of patients are affected)
- IgA deficiency (prevalence increased tenfold).

Is the incidence of coeliac disease changing?

Several studies have evaluated the incidence of coeliac disease retrospectively. The results have been conflicting, because only the visible part of the coeliac iceberg has been considered. A multicentre European survey reported widely different incidence rates per 1000 births ranging from 0.078 in Greece to 3.51 in Sweden. These results, rather than reflecting true differences in the prevalence of coeliac disease, could be the result of:

- differences in the intake of gluten-containing cereals, particularly during infancy (Figure 2.4); this could, in turn, modify the clinical expression of coeliac disease and the probability that the disorder will be correctly diagnosed
- varying degrees of awareness of coeliac disease among doctors; 'you will find coeliac disease only if you think of it' is an aphorism worth remembering.

During the 1980s, a rising incidence of coeliac disease was reported in several European countries, which was generally associated with an increase in the

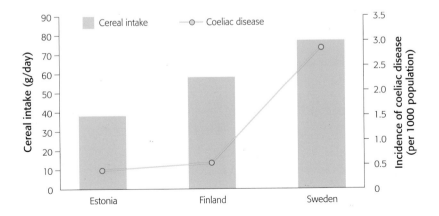

Figure 2.4 The intake of gluten-containing cereals during infancy is related to some extent to the incidence of coeliac disease in these neighbouring countries. Data from Mitt and Uibo 1998.

mean age at diagnosis. This is easily explained by the availability of powerful screening tests for coeliac disease, which allowed the recognition of many atypical, late-onset forms that would previously have been overlooked.

Is mass screening for coeliac disease worthwhile?

Coeliac disease would appear to fulfil the criteria for mass screening.

- It is a potentially serious condition that produces significant morbidity.
- Early clinical detection is often difficult.
- If not recognized early, it can present with severe complications, such as malignancy, osteoporosis and neurological problems, which are difficult to manage.
- A GFD is an effective therapy.
- Sensitive, simple and cheap screening tests are available.

However, the time for mass coeliac disease screening has not yet come, as important pieces of information are still lacking. A deeper understanding of the natural history of the condition is urgently needed to ascertain the

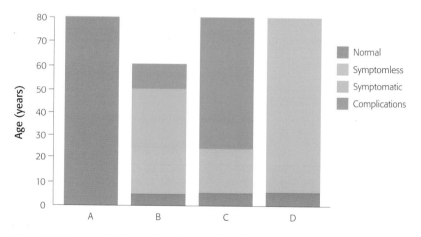

Figure 2.5 The natural history of undiagnosed coeliac disease in three patients (B, C and D) compared with a healthy control (A). A pre-clinical diagnosis might have been useful in the case of patient B, who had a shorter lifespan due to the onset of an intestinal lymphoma, and in patient C, who experienced neurological complications impairing the quality of life. An early diagnosis would be of no benefit, and may possibly be detrimental, in individuals with true silent coeliac disease who have a normal duration and quality of life, such as patient D.

outcome in the many affected individuals who escape a clinical diagnosis and to determine whether they are susceptible to the complications affecting those patients diagnosed clinically. A programme of case finding is a better option at the present time; that is, doctors should be alert to the possibility of coeliac disease in patients who present with ill health or in whom tests indicate that the disorder may be present.

The concept of lead time is central to the rationale of disease control by early detection and treatment. The lead time is the interval between detection and the time at which the diagnosis would have been made without screening. The lead-time duration and the distribution of lead times among affected individuals are not known for coeliac disease. Should patients have an indefinitely long lead time due to non-progressive preclinical disease, mass screening would be of no benefit and may even be detrimental because of the psychosocial effects of a GFD (Figure 2.5).

CHAPTER 3

Pathophysiology

Coeliac disease is a multifactorial disorder that depends on both genetic and environmental factors for expression. The disease appears to be specific to man and the lack of an animal model has hampered research. Although the pathogenesis of coeliac disease is not yet completely understood, there is evidence to suggest that it is an autoimmune disorder triggered and maintained by an external antigen, namely gluten, in the diet.

Gluten

The term gluten is generically applied to a family of storage proteins found in wheat, rye and barley (8–14% by weight) (Figure 3.1). All the proteins that are harmful to patients with coeliac disease are rich in proline and

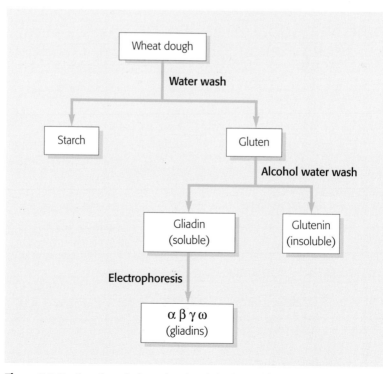

Figure 3.1 Fractionation of wheat showing derivation of gluten and gliadin.

glutamine, and are collectively called prolamins. The prolamin fractions of the various cereals carry different names; gliadin (wheat), secalin (rye) and hordein (barley). The prolamins of oats (avenin) account for only 5–15% of the total seed protein, which could partly explain why coeliac patients may tolerate oats in the diet. The major coeliac toxic protein is gliadin, which comprises about 50% of wheat proteins. In a single wheat variety, there are approximately 45 different gliadins, which can be subdivided into α, β, γ and ω subfractions according to their electrophoretic mobility. This complexity has made gluten a difficult substance to investigate within the context of coeliac disease.

The sequence of A-gliadin, a protein made up of 266 amino acids, has been determined. Peptides derived from A-gliadin have been shown to have damaging effects in coeliac disease by *in-vitro* and *in-vivo* studies (e.g. the peptide corresponding to amino acid residues 31–49). It has been hypothesized that the peptide QQQPFP (where Q represents glutamine, P, proline and F, phenylalanine) could be one of the core specific sequences of toxic prolamins.

A similarity between part of the A-gliadin sequence and the E1b coat protein of the human adenovirus type 12 (Ad 12) has been noted. Although the role of Ad 12 in the pathogenesis of coeliac disease has not been confirmed by experimental data, this hypothesis points towards a possible process of molecular mimicry between viral and gliadin proteins that could, in turn, activate the immune system and trigger coeliac disease in susceptible individuals.

Jejunal mucosa

Abnormalities of the jejunal mucosa are the hallmark of coeliac disease. The diagnosis is based on characteristic appearances of the enterocytes, villi, crypts and the inflammatory cell infiltrate in the mucosa.

Normal mucosa. Digitate villi, leaf forms and ridges are seen in normal jejunal mucosa (Figures 3.2a and 3.3a). When viewed by transmission light microscopy, the villi constitute 65–80% of the total mucosal thickness, while the crypts make up the remainder (Figure 3.4). The villi are covered by a single layer of columnar cells called enterocytes, which have a basally situated nucleus and a well-marked brush border. Cells migrate up the crypts to replace enterocytes, which are being continually lost from the villous tips into the bowel lumen. In the epithelium, the sparse cellular infiltrate is made up almost exclusively of IEL, while in the lamina propria, it is composed mainly of plasma cells, lymphocytes and macrophages.

Coeliac mucosa. The mucosa appears flat with a mosaic pattern under the light-dissecting microscope (Figure 3.2b). Histologically, there are no structures in the mucosa that can be identified as villi (Figure 3.5). The crypts are hypertrophied and open directly on to the mucosal surface.

(a)

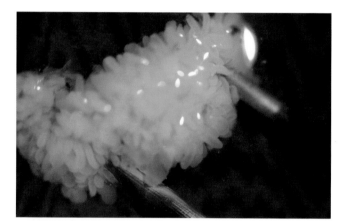

(b)

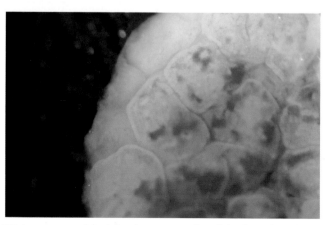

Figure 3.2 Appearance of the jejunal mucosa under a light-dissecting microscope. (a) Normal mucosa showing finger-like villi. (b) The flat mucosa of coeliac disease showing the characteristic mosaic appearance.

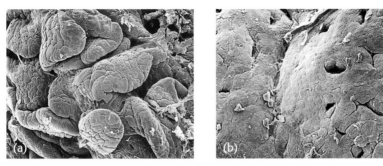

Figure 3.3 Appearance of the jejunal mucosa under the scanning electron microscope. (a) Normal mucosa with leaf-shaped villi protruding into the intestinal lumen (x 100). (b) The typical flat mucosa and crater-shaped openings of the crypts in untreated coeliac disease (x 150). Reproduced courtesy of S Cinti and M Morroni of the Morphology Institute of Ancona University, Ancona.

The cells constituting the mucosal surface are cuboidal and appear stratified, and the brush border is poorly developed. A dense infiltrate of lymphocytes and plasma cells is found in the lamina propria and the IEL are increased in number. The openings of the crypts directly on to the surface of the mucosa are shown particularly well by scanning electron microscopy (Figure 3.3b). Although a number of other conditions may cause a flat biopsy (Table 3.1), such findings in an adult living in the western world are almost certain to indicate coeliac disease.

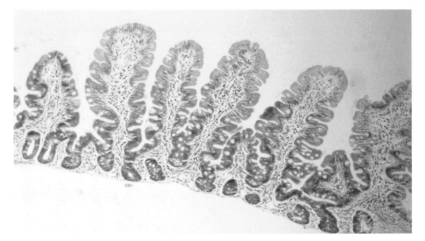

Figure 3.4 Normal jejunal mucosa showing digitate villi.

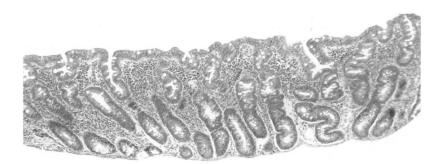

Figure 3.5 Jejunal biopsy from a patient with untreated coeliac disease. Villi are absent and the crypts hypertrophied. Intraepithelial lymphocytes are increased in number and a heavy infiltrate of plasma cells and lymphocytes is evident in the lamina propria.

Spectrum of gluten sensitivity and mucosal pathology

Recently, it has become clear from observations made in patients with dermatitis herpetiformis and in relatives of patients with coeliac disease, as well as from gluten-challenge studies, that the classical appearances of coeliac disease form only one facet of gluten sensitivity and that less severe lesions can occur. Thus, a structurally normal mucosa but bearing an increased density of

TABLE 3.1

Conditions causing a flat jejunal mucosa

• Coeliac disease	• Refractory sprue
• Collagenous sprue	• Cows' milk protein intolerance
• Soy protein intolerance	• Immunodeficiency syndromes
• Mediterranean lymphoma	• Intestinal ulceration
• Gastroenteritis	• Intractable diarrhoea of infancy
• Protein calorie malnutrition	• Kwashiorkor
• Tropical sprue	• Parasitic infections
• Human immunodeficiency virus	• Bowel ischaemia
• Eosinophilic gastroenteritis	• Contaminated bowel syndrome
• Autoimmune enteropathy	• Drug and radiation damage

IEL expressing γ/δ T cell receptors, and aberrant HLA-DR expression in crypt epithelial cells, falls within the gluten sensitivity spectrum. Further support for this comes from observations of changes in the mucosa as coeliac disease evolves. Patients may initially have near-normal biopsies that later become flat, and may have increased serum AGA concentrations, and more importantly AEA, which is further evidence of gluten sensitivity.

The typical flat mucosa found in active coeliac disease is likely to be the end-stage lesion of T-cell-dependent immune reactivity that progresses through several phases (Figure 3.6):

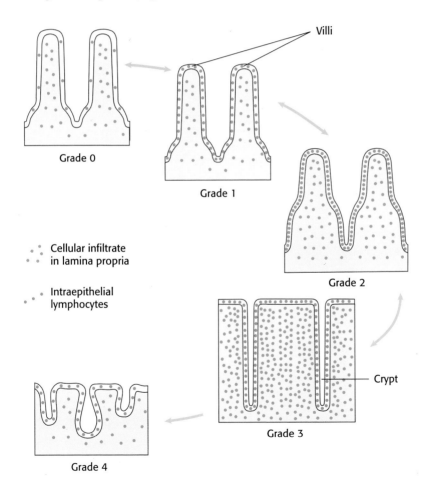

Figure 3.6 Grading of mucosal lesions associated with gluten sensitivity.

- a less severe infiltrative lesion characterized by isolated infiltration of IEL, especially CD8+ T lymphocytes, within a structurally normal mucosa (Grade 1)
- a hyperplastic lesion showing crypt hypertrophy (Grade 2)
- a flat/destructive lesion with the greatly hypertrophied crypts and the characteristically flattened villi (Grade 3).

There is a dynamic relationship between these grades with progression in either direction. An important factor influencing the severity of the enteropathy is the amount of gluten ingested, but other factors include gastrointestinal infections and the stresses of surgery or pregnancy. The mucosal pathology of gluten sensitivity and coeliac disease is even wider than this, as some patients with dermatitis herpetiformis have biopsies that appear indistinguishable from normal (Grade 0), and an irreversible, atrophic lesion (Grade 4) associated with jejunoileitis and enteropathy-associated T-cell lymphoma (EATL) also occurs.

Extent of disease. Although coeliac enteropathy is typically confined to the duodenum and proximal jejunum, the length of the damaged intestine is variable. The residual unaffected bowel could undergo functional hypertrophy and thus determine the balance between clinical 'silence' and symptoms. This possibility has recently been confirmed by a dual sugar intestinal permeability study. Children with typical coeliac disease usually show a decrease in mannitol urinary recovery, which is thought to reflect the decrease in the overall intestinal mucosa surface. Individuals with silent coeliac disease, however, have a mannitol urinary recovery within normal limits (Figure 3.7), which suggests that they remain symptom-free because the damaged area of intestinal mucosa is small.

Immunohistological features

Coeliac enteropathy is most likely the result of immune-mediated damage to the small intestinal mucosa. The structural and immunohistological features of the coeliac enteropathy closely resemble those seen in animal models of T-cell mucosal injury, such as allograft rejection, graft-versus-host disease or experimental giardiasis.

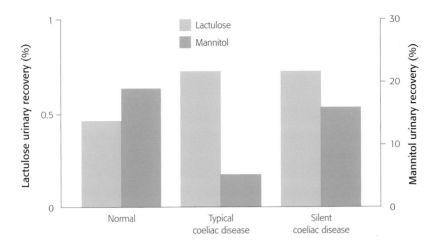

Figure 3.7 The results of the lactulose/mannitol intestinal permeability test suggest a possible explanation for the different expressions of coeliac disease. Lactulose urinary recovery (which may reflect paracellular permeability) is increased in both typical and silent forms of the disease due to the presence of enteropathy. However, mannitol recovery (which is directly related to the absorptive surface area) is reduced only in typical forms. This indicates that the mucosal damage extends for a shorter distance down the bowel in clinically silent cases.

Tissue transglutaminase. Recently, tissue transglutaminase (tTG), a ubiquitous enzyme that catalyses the cross-linking of proteins, has been reported to be the autoantigen responsible for the positivity of AEA. Interestingly, gliadin is an excellent substrate for tTG because of its high glutamine content (about 40%). These findings support the autoimmune theory for a number of reasons.

- Damage to the intestinal epithelium, caused either by toxic fractions of gluten or other agents (e.g. viruses), might trigger the extracellular release of cytosolic tTG, mainly by lamina propria mesenchymal cells.
- Gliadin is deamidated by tTG with subsequent formation of gliadin–tTG complexes.
- Neo-epitopes could then initiate an immune response in genetically predisposed individuals, directed both to gliadin and tTG.

T-lymphocyte activation. At least two separate signals are required to activate T lymphocytes. One is the recognition of antigen by specific T-cell clones. The other is common to most T cells and involves co-stimulation of the CD28 molecule found on the cell surface by CD80 (B7.1) and/or CD86 (B7.2), expressed on antigen-presenting cells. CTLA-4 immuno-globulin (CTLA-4Ig) disrupts the activation of CD28 and so leads to T-cell tolerance. Animal experiments have shown that CTLA-4Ig will prolong grafts and suppress immune-mediated disorders. In an organ culture system, CTLA-4Ig suppressed interleukin 2 (IL-2), interferon γ (IFN-γ), CD25 and intercellular adhesion molecule 1 (ICAM-1) positive cells in the lamina propria of small intestinal biopsies from patients with treated coeliac disease challenged *in vitro* with gliadin. In addition, production of epithelial membrane antigen by biopsies was suppressed and apoptosis of T cells induced. These results suggest that CTLA-4Ig might be of value in the treatment of coeliac disease and developments are eagerly awaited. Interestingly, however, CTLA-4Ig does not appear to influence T-cell migration in the epithelium of the small intestine in coeliac disease or affect enterocyte *Fas* expression, which indicates that factors other than T lymphocytes are necessary in the pathogenesis of the disease.

Cytokines. Intestinal cytokine responses in the small intestinal mucosa, as determined by mRNA expression, indicate that gluten induces a rapid increase in IFN-γ as well as low levels of IL-2, IL-4, IL-6 and tumour necrosis factor γ (TNF-γ). These events develop in the lamina propria. IFN-γ mRNA is increased by about a 1000-fold in untreated coeliac disease compared with controls. IFN-γ causes damage to small bowel mucosa and this can be blocked by anti-IFN-γ antibody. A greater understanding of the role of cytokines might lead to new therapies for coeliac disease.

Pathophysiological pathway. A possible pathophysiological pathway leading to tissue damage in coeliac disease is illustrated in Figure 3.8. The products of HLA genes are proteins located on the membrane of antigen-presenting cells (e.g. macrophages). The HLA molecule forms a 'groove' in which short peptides (e.g. products of gliadin digestion) can be specifically linked. Deamidation of gliadin by tTG unmasks neo-epitopes that efficiently bind to HLA-DQ2 molecules on antigen-presenting cells. The interaction between gliadin peptides and HLA molecules activates intestinal T cells via the T-cell receptor. The release of pro-inflammatory cytokines (e.g. IFN-γ, TNF-α,

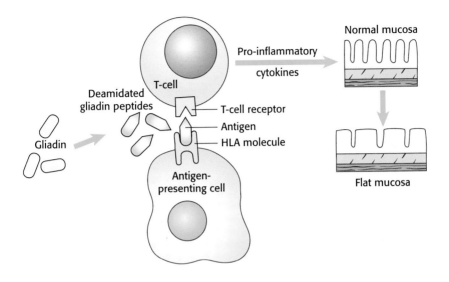

Figure 3.8 A possible pathway leading to intestinal mucosal damage in coeliac disease. Gliadin peptides (after deamidation by tissue transglutaminase) are presented by antigen-presenting cells to T lymphocytes (T cells). The antigen is held in a groove formed by the human leucocyte antigen (HLA) molecule and the complex is recognized by the T cell. This activates the T cell and pro-inflammatory cytokines are produced. These may damage the enterocytes and thereby the mucosa, either directly or via the intraepithelial lymphocytes.

IL-2) by activated T cells could damage enterocytes, increase cellular proliferation in the intestinal crypts and lead to the flat mucosal lesion characteristic of coeliac disease.

CHAPTER 4

Clinical manifestations

Coeliac disease presents with a wide spectrum of clinical manifestations. The diagnosis will often be overlooked unless it is actively considered in patients with unexplained clinical and laboratory features in whom it is a possibility (Table 4.1).

Factors affecting clinical presentation

The reasons why the clinical expression of coeliac disease is so highly variable and why presentation can occur at any time in life, from infancy to very old age, are not fully understood. A number of factors have, however, been implicated.

Age. The symptoms of malabsorption are usually more marked during the first years of life and then gradually decrease. This is probably due to the decreasing ratio between the length of the diseased proximal and the unaffected distal small intestine.

TABLE 4.1

Features suggestive of coeliac disease

- History of coeliac disease in childhood
- Recurrent abdominal pain in childhood
- Delayed puberty
- Short stature
- Old rickets
- Non-specific ill health
- Weight loss
- Diarrhoea
- Malabsorption syndrome
- Recurrent aphthous mouth ulcers

- Anaemia, raised mean corpuscular volume, folate and iron deficiency
- Hypocalcaemia
- Osteoporosis and osteomalacia
- Infertility and recurrent miscarriages
- IgA deficiency
- Splenic atrophy and hyposplenism
- Abnormal International Normalized Ratio (INR)
- Unexplained neurological disturbances
- Unexplained hypertransaminasaemia

Amount of ingested gluten. The probability that a patient will have a severe enteropathy, and therefore the clinical manifestations of coeliac disease, increases with the amount of gluten that is eaten. In Sweden, most infants with coeliac disease become symptomatic during the first 2 years of life because Swedish weaning food contains a large quantity of wheat flour.

Intestinal infections. The absorptive defect caused by coeliac disease in the proximal small intestine can be masked by compensation in the distal ileum. The diffuse impairment of intestinal function caused by an intestinal infection can precipitate the onset of diarrhoea and unmask coeliac disease.

Pregnancy. Occasionally, coeliac disease becomes clinically manifest during pregnancy or soon after childbirth.

Surgery. The stress of an operation (e.g. partial gastrectomy or hysterectomy) can precipitate symptoms of coeliac disease.

Lymphoma. The development of intestinal lymphoma may unmask coeliac disease.

Presentation in children and adolescents

Typical coeliac disease. The typical child presents between 6 and 24 months of age with impaired growth, abnormal stools, abdominal distension, muscle wasting and hypotonia, poor appetite and unhappy behaviour (Figure 4.1); pallor and oedema may also be seen. The onset of symptoms is gradual and usually characterized by a time lag of some months after weaning. Weight gain velocity slowly decreases and weight loss then follows (Figure 4.2). The stools become frequent, pale, soft, bulky and offensive. Occasionally, constipation is a prominent feature. Vomiting commonly occurs in very young infants.

When diagnostic facilities are not readily available (e.g. in some developing countries), long-standing, untreated coeliac disease is characterized by stunting, pubertal delay, chronic diarrhoea, abdominal distension and severe iron deficiency anaemia.

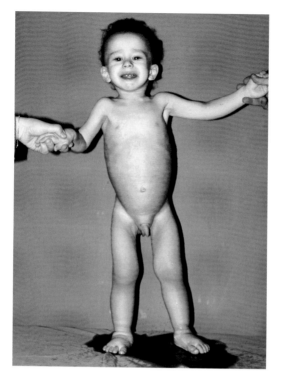

Figure 4.1 A child aged 15 months with typical coeliac disease. He is irritable and severely malnourished with abdominal distension and oedema.

Figure 4.2 The 'parabolic' weight curve of a child with typical coeliac disease. The child gained weight following the introduction of a gluten-free diet.

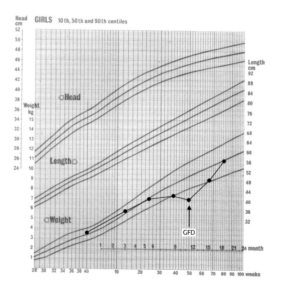

Atypical coeliac disease is usually seen in older children and features of overt malabsorption are absent. The symptoms and signs may be intestinal or extraintestinal.

Intestinal features may include:
- recurrent abdominal pain
- dental enamel defects (Figure 4.3)
- recurrent aphthous stomatitis
- cryptogenic hepatitis.

Extraintestinal features. Between 6 and 12% of patients with iron deficiency anaemia attending a haematology clinic are found to have coeliac disease; the anaemia is often resistant to oral iron therapy.

Short stature and delayed puberty can be the primary manifestation in an otherwise healthy child. Coeliac disease is the most common organic cause of slow height velocity and is more common than growth hormone deficiency. The endocrinological pattern includes delayed bone age, normal growth hormone response to stimulatory tests, normal levels of insulin-like growth factor-1 (IGF-1) and decreased serum levels of IGF-binding protein 3. Treatment with a GFD usually leads to complete catch-up growth within 2–3 years.

Coeliac disease can also present with joint disease. This takes the form of pain and stiffness affecting mainly shoulders, elbows, knees and hands.

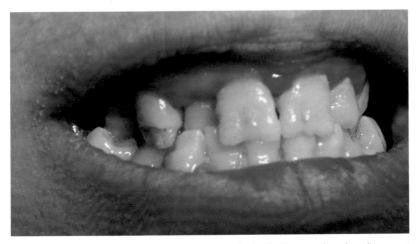

Figure 4.3 Dental enamel defects in a patient with newly diagnosed coeliac disease. Reproduced courtesy of A Ventura, University Department of Paediatrics, Trieste, Italy.

Symptoms may improve or disappear on a GFD. The deposition of immune complexes in the joints may produce these symptoms.

Silent coeliac disease. Since the introduction of serological screening tests, silent coeliac disease has been increasingly recognized. A thorough history and investigation will, however, reveal a low-grade illness in many of these individuals. Common features are:
- behavioural disturbances, such as depression, irritability and impaired school performance
- impaired physical fitness and easily fatigued
- iron deficiency with or without anaemia
- reduced bone mineral density.

Adolescents with coeliac disease, who are detected by screening and are apparently healthy at diagnosis, usually report improved physical and psychological well-being following gluten withdrawal. The most common changes are increased height and weight velocity, increased appetite, mood amelioration, and increased physical and school performance.

Presentation in adults

Patients with overt malabsorption and severe symptoms of coeliac disease are still seen, but most now present with trivial or non-specific complaints. The diagnosis is often only suspected from abnormalities found on routine blood tests, particularly anaemia, a raised mean corpuscular volume (MCV), iron and folate deficiency, and hypocalcaemia which, together with hypophosphataemia and elevated alkaline phosphatase, indicates osteomalacia. Some cases are identified from family studies or screening programmes. While many patients consider themselves to have mild or even no symptoms, they are often only able to recognize the full extent of their ill health retrospectively, following the benefits conferred by a GFD. Many will find that they had accepted a significant degree of illness as normal. Thus, as in paediatric practice, adults may present with typical or atypical symptoms, or with silent coeliac disease.

Clinical features. The features of coeliac disease at presentation are protean (Table 4.2 and Figure 4.4). Diarrhoea is the most common symptom, but only affects just over 50% of patients, is of variable duration (40% of patients < 1 year and 35% < 5 years) and can present acutely in a previously

TABLE 4.2
Presenting features of coeliac disease

General

- Short stature
- Weight loss
- Lassitude/lethargy
- Oedema
- Clubbing
- Koilonychia
- Bruising

Gastrointestinal

- Anorexia, nausea, vomiting
- Glossitis, mouth ulcers
- Abdominal distension and pain
- Flatulence and flatus
- Diarrhoea, constipation

Psychiatric

- Depression
- Anxiety

Neurological

- Peripheral neuropathy
- Ataxia
- Epilepsy

Haematological

- Anaemia
- Folic acid and iron deficiency
- Raised mean corpuscular volume
- Haemorrhagic manifestations

Biochemical

- Reduced serum calcium, raised alkaline phosphatase
- Hypertransaminasaemia

Reproduction

- Infertility
- Recurrent miscarriages

Musculoskeletal

- Osteomalacia, osteoporosis, bone pain
- Myopathy
- Cramps, tetany, paraesthesia

Renal

- Nocturnal diuresis

Skin

- Dermatitis herpetiformis
- Pigmentation

well person. Lethargy and tiredness, with or without anaemia or other features, and weight loss are also common symptoms. Abdominal distension affects about one-third of patients. Peripheral neuropathy, ataxia indicating spinocerebellar degeneration, arthropathy, infertility and bleeding disorders are less common presentations. In about 4% of cases, coeliac disease presents during pregnancy or within weeks or months of giving birth. It is noteworthy that only about 5% of patients are asymptomatic if a careful history is elicited, but in about one-third of patients, there are no abnormal signs.

(a)

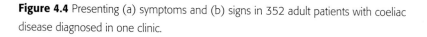

Figure 4.4 Presenting (a) symptoms and (b) signs in 352 adult patients with coeliac disease diagnosed in one clinic.

The elderly. Coeliac disease is being increasingly diagnosed in later life and, today, about 25% of cases are diagnosed in patients over 60 years of age (Table 4.3 and Figure 4.5). Contrary to common belief, 95% of these patients manage a GFD well and enjoy a much improved quality of life.

TABLE 4.3

Age at which patients joined the Coeliac Society in the UK*

Age (years)	1994	1997
Under 15	455	455
16–59	2002	2673
60–85+	532	1062
Total number of members	2989	4190

*It is assumed that the date of joining is close to the date of diagnosis. Reproduced with permission from the Coeliac Society (UK)

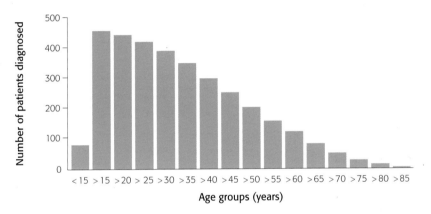

Figure 4.5 Age of patients with coeliac disease at diagnosis attending the Derby Adult Coeliac Clinic.

Associated disorders

Many disorders occur in association with coeliac disease, which can cause diagnostic difficulties if the clinical features are attributed to the established diagnosis rather than prompt a search for a second diagnosis.

Disturbed immunity in coeliac disease may predispose affected individuals to other disorders that also have an immunological aetiology. The disorders most commonly associated with coeliac disease are:

- type 1 diabetes mellitus
- autoimmune liver disease
- thyroid disorders
- pulmonary diseases, such as fibrosing alveolitis and asthma

33

- ulcerative colitis
- Crohn's disease
- Sjögren's syndrome
- parathyroid disorders
- IgA deficiency.

There may be an association with Down's syndrome and cystic fibrosis. Although patients may have joint and neurological disturbances, it is not clear whether specific disorders occur in coeliac disease.

The development of reliable screening tests and the use of endoscopy to obtain small bowel biopsies has made diagnosis of associated coeliac disease much easier. For example, in one study, diabetic patients were screened using AGA, followed by duodenal biopsy. Approximately 2% of patients were found to have coeliac disease; 50% of these had symptoms attributable to coeliac disease that improved with a GFD.

Dermatitis herpetiformis

Dermatitis herpetiformis is part of the spectrum of coeliac disease and is discussed in Chapter 8.

Failure to respond to a gluten-free diet

The concept of non-responsive coeliac disease has generated much debate. If coeliac disease is defined as a condition that responds to a GFD in terms of symptoms and the morphology of the small bowel mucosa then, by definition, coeliac disease is not present if there is no response. If, however, a less restrictive definition is used and the criterion for diagnosis is a flat mucosa, irrespective of the response to a GFD, then non-responsiveness can be accepted. In any event, 10–15% of patients continue to have symptoms on a GFD and require assessment, while others may respond symptomatically to diet, but still have a flat or severely damaged mucosa. A number of factors need to be considered in these patients.

- Continued ingestion of gluten, either inadvertently or on purpose, is the most common reason for non-responsiveness; measurement of AGA can be helpful in such cases.
- Other foods may be implicated (e.g. milk, eggs, chicken, tuna, soy) and health improves when these are also excluded from the diet.
- Replacement of trace elements (e.g. zinc) may be beneficial.

- There may be bacterial overgrowth in the jejunum.
- Pancreatic insufficiency can occur.
- A malignancy, particularly lymphoma, may have developed.
- There may be chronic ulceration in the small bowel.
- Mesenteric lymph node cavitation can occur.
- Other disorders (e.g. ulcerative colitis or Crohn's disease) may be present.

CHAPTER 5

Diagnosis

A high index of clinical suspicion is essential to identify patients with coeliac disease. Once the possibility has been recognized, tests should be carried out to confirm the diagnosis (Table 5.1). If complications of malignancy or bowel ulceration are suspected at presentation, additional investigations will be required.

Blood tests

Haematological and biochemical profiles should be obtained for all patients whenever possible.

- Anaemia is often present and should not be overlooked even when it is mild. Measurement of serum ferritin, folate and vitamin B_{12} will help to establish the cause of the anaemia. Folate and ferritin deficiencies are common and, while low concentrations of vitamin B_{12} are often found, pernicious anaemia is rare in coeliac disease.
- A low or elevated MCV sometimes occurs in the absence of anaemia and reflects deficiencies of iron (low MCV), folate and vitamin B_{12} (high MCV).
- If features of hyposplenism (e.g. Howell-Jolly bodies, thrombocytosis) are present, coeliac disease is the most likely cause if the patient has not had a splenectomy.
- Pancytopenia is uncommon and is usually due to folate or vitamin B_{12} deficiency.

TABLE 5.1

Tests to confirm a diagnosis of coeliac disease

- Routine blood tests and the measurement of specific indices
- Biopsy of the small intestinal mucosa
- Serological markers
- Tests of intestinal absorption
- Imaging

- A prolonged prothrombin time due to vitamin K deficiency is rare, but should be corrected before taking a small bowel biopsy.
- Lymphocytopenia may be present and probably reflects the lymphoid atrophy associated with coeliac disease.
- Hypocalcaemia, hypophosphataemia and elevated alkaline phosphatase indicate osteomalacia. Hypocalcaemia may, however, occur as an isolated finding.
- Mild elevation of aminotransferases (aspartate and alanine) may occur in coeliac disease.
- Mild hypoalbuminaemia may be present, and may reflect increased protein loss in the gut and reduced liver synthesis. Marked hypoalbuminaemia indicates severe malabsorption or the presence of complications, such as lymphoma or bowel ulcerations.
- IgA deficiency can be seen; coeliac disease is ten times more common in IgA-deficient individuals than in the general population.

Biopsy of small intestinal mucosa

The diagnosis of coeliac disease has centred on the appearance of the jejunal mucosa, and the responses to gluten withdrawal and challenge, and associated clinical reactions. As understanding has increased, the concept of silent, latent and potential coeliac disease has emerged, which, together with the development of serological tests, has made it necessary to re-evaluate the diagnostic criteria. Small intestinal biopsy is, however, still the cornerstone of diagnosis and should be undertaken in all patients with suspected coeliac disease.

Obtaining biopsies. Biopsies can be obtained using a capsule with a suction-guillotine mechanism (e.g. Crosby capsule, Watson capsule). Nowadays, most biopsies in adults are taken at the time of upper gastrointestinal endoscopy using standard fibre-optic instruments. Endoscopy allows multiple biopsies to be taken, which minimizes sampling error, and in many patients, views of the mucosa will support or refute the diagnosis even before the results of the biopsies are available.

Larger biopsies taken by capsules can be orientated and placed on card to be inspected under the dissecting microscope, which will differentiate normal and flat specimens. The smaller biopsies obtained at endoscopy should be placed floating free in formalin for processing by the pathology laboratory; attempts to orientate the sample often results in damage that makes interpretation difficult or impossible.

Enteroscopy has the potential to enable biopsies to be obtained further down the duodenum and the small bowel to be examined for ulcerations, carcinomas and lymphomas. This technique is still being evaluated, but may have a small role in the investigation of patients with suspected complications. Enteroscopy does, however, carry the risk of intestinal perforation.

Diagnosis in children

In 1969, the European Society of Paediatric Gastroenterology laid down criteria for the diagnosis of coeliac disease in children. This entailed three biopsies showing:

- an initial flat mucosa in the upper small intestine
- restoration of the mucosa to normal on a GFD
- deterioration of the mucosa after gluten challenge.

With increased knowledge, these criteria have been modified. Only if a gluten challenge is carried out will the second and third biopsies be performed, but this is not now considered necessary in all patients. Some believe that a second biopsy to check mucosal recovery should always be carried out, because many children are asymptomatic and improvement cannot be monitored clinically, while others who do not fully comply with the GFD may appear well, but have mucosal abnormalities.

Diagnosis in adults

Opinions as to how the diagnosis should be established in adults have also differed. An initial biopsy is mandatory. A flat biopsy from a patient in the western world almost certainly indicates coeliac disease and many would accept the diagnosis based on this criterion. Some require a clinical response to gluten withdrawal to make the diagnosis, but this cannot be used in those who do not have symptoms. Others require demonstration of an improvement in the appearance of the mucosa, but in practice, while continuing abnormality may indicate laxity with the diet, it seldom changes the diagnosis.

Gluten challenge

Gluten challenge is a provocation test performed to confirm the diagnosis of coeliac disease and is particularly useful in children. After the patient has been treated with a GFD for 12–24 months, a jejunal biopsy is taken to confirm a return to normal histology. Gluten is then re-introduced either as a fixed daily amount (e.g. 5 g) or as free intake of gluten-containing products. A further biopsy is performed when either symptoms of relapse appear or after 3–6 months. Deterioration of the mucosal architecture confirms the persistence of gluten intolerance and the patient is returned to a GFD. Since gluten challenge confirms the initial diagnosis in most cases (> 95%) and can be a distressing experience, it is now considered necessary only in selected cases. These include:

- when there is doubt about the initial diagnosis (e.g. no initial biopsy), or the biopsy was inadequate or not characteristic of coeliac disease
- children diagnosed during the first 2 years of life, because other causes of enteropathy resembling coeliac disease (e.g. cows' milk intolerance) are common at this age
- teenagers who intend to abandon the GFD in a controlled way.

Gluten challenge should not be undertaken before the age of 6 years to avoid dental damage.

In adults, gluten challenge has very little place. It is used occasionally to confirm the diagnosis in patients who started a GFD before a biopsy was taken.

Transient gluten intolerance

Transient gluten intolerance has been described in young children who are usually less than 2 years of age at the time of the initial diagnosis and who show:

- an initial illness associated with a severe small intestinal enteropathy
- complete clinical remission on a GFD
- normal intestinal mucosa 2 years or more after a return to a gluten-containing diet.

Transient gluten intolerance is regarded as a rare condition that should be included in the broad group of food protein sensitive enteropathies of infancy.

The wide application of gluten challenge for confirmation of the diagnosis of coeliac disease has enlivened the debate on transient gluten intolerance and whether it really exists. It has been shown that, in a few patients, it can be

9–14 years before a flat mucosa develops on gluten challenge. Patients suspected of transient gluten intolerance should, therefore, undergo long-term follow up, with repeated intestinal biopsies, as it is possible that some of them will have coeliac disease and have a late relapse.

Serological markers of coeliac disease

If coeliac disease is strongly suspected from the clinical features and laboratory findings, an intestinal biopsy is required to confirm or refute the diagnosis, and antibody tests are unnecessary. These investigations have a place:

- if the probability of coeliac disease is low; a negative antibody test will avoid a biopsy
- in screening groups at particular risk of coeliac disease, but who do not have overt features (e.g. relatives of patients with coeliac disease, patients with type 1 diabetes mellitus)
- in monitoring compliance with a GFD (Figure 5.1)

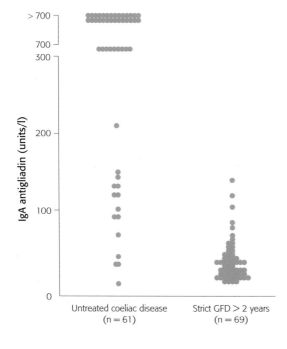

Figure 5.1 Monitoring adherence to a gluten-free diet (GFD) with antigliadin antibodies (AGA). Of 61 patients with untreated coeliac disease, only 5 had concentrations of IgA AGA within the normal range (< 90 units/litre), one of whom was IgA deficient. The results for almost all of the 69 patients treated with a GFD for more than 2 years were within the normal range.

- in the diagnosis of coeliac disease in children; monitoring antibodies after gluten challenge may avoid further biopsies.

It is important to remember that IgA class antibodies are not generated by IgA-deficient individuals and care must be taken in interpreting the results. In these patients, IgG class antibodies may be measured.

Antigliadin antibodies were the first serological markers of coeliac disease to be widely used in clinical practice. They were introduced in the early 1980s and a number of commercial kits are now available. The IgA-class AGA, measured using ELISA, has a sensitivity of 75–93% and a high specificity (> 95%). Although some have recommended the use of both IgA- and IgG-class AGA, the poor specificity of the IgG AGA (80%) leads to many false-positive results and unnecessary endoscopic biopsies. IgA AGA is the most useful marker in symptomatic children under 2 years of age. AGA results are usually given in arbitrary units that differ depending on the kit used, but one assay expresses results as ng/ml of specific antibody.

If gliadin gains access to the immune system through 'leaky' mucous membranes, antibodies will be produced. Raised levels may, therefore, also be found in a number of other conditions (Table 5.2); AEA are not detected in these disorders.

Antiendomysial antibodies are autoantibodies directed against antigens in the collagenous matrix of human and monkey tissues. The usual method for detecting IgA AEA is indirect immunofluorescence with sections of either monkey oesophagus or human umbilical cord (Figure 5.2). For ethical reasons, human umbilical cord is currently considered the substrate of

TABLE 5.2

Common causes of false-positive antigliadin antibody tests

• Oesophagitis	• Gastritis
• Recent gastroenteritis	• Cows' milk protein allergy
• Ulcerative colitis	• Crohn's disease
• Cystic fibrosis	• Rheumatoid arthritis
• Down's syndrome	

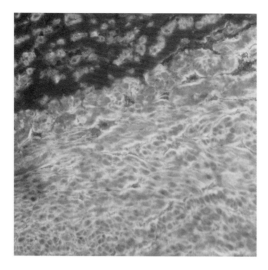

Figure 5.2 Indirect immunofluorescence staining pattern for antiendomysial antibody using human umbilical cord exposed to serum from a patient with untreated coeliac disease. The positivity is seen around the smooth muscle fibres of the vessels as a honeycomb reticular network.

choice, although the immunofluorescence pattern with this substrate is not always easy to interpret. The specificity of this test approaches 100%; false-positive results are extremely rare or even non-existent. Early claims of 100% sensitivity for the AEA test have been disputed but, in some recent series, figures of about 90% have been obtained; thus, the diagnosis could be missed if this were the only test to be used. False-negative results can be obtained in children less than 2 years of age.

AEA are produced by biopsies from untreated coeliac patients and from treated patients challenged *in vitro* with gliadin. This refinement may form the basis of a further test for coeliac disease.

Antireticulin antibodies (ARA) are antibodies that react against extracellular connective tissue fibrils (reticulin). They are detected by indirect immunofluorescence using rodent substrates (e.g. liver). ARA and AEA are probably the same autoantibody, but detected on different substrates. However, AEA are preferred in the diagnosis of active coeliac disease because of their superior sensitivity.

Anti-tissue transglutaminase antibodies. Recently, tTG has been reported to be the putative autoantigen responsible for AEA positivity in coeliac disease. An ELISA method has been developed for the determination of anti-tTG autoantibodies, which could replace the AEA assay in the future.

Tests of intestinal absorption

Faecal fat measurement. Steatorrhoea can be shown by microscopy.
The number of fat globules greatly increases after the slides are heated.
In experienced hands, this is a simple and useful investigation, but it can
be misleading. The measurement of fat is now obsolete and has no part to
play in the diagnosis of coeliac disease, because many patients do not have
steatorrhoea and better tests are available.

Serum carotene. Low serum levels of carotene are commonly found in coeliac
patients, particularly young children, because of malabsorption of fat-soluble
vitamins.

Intestinal permeability. The D-xylose absorption test is no longer used to
measure the integrity of the mucosa because it is unreliable. Permeability is
now assessed using differential sugar absorption. This test is performed by
measuring the urinary recovery of two sugars of different molecular sizes and
different absorption routes after oral administration, such as lactulose and
mannitol (Figure 5.3). In untreated coeliac disease, increased urinary excretion
of lactulose (due to increased paracellular enterocyte permeability) associated
with decreased mannitol recovery (because of reduced intestinal mucosal

(a)   (b)

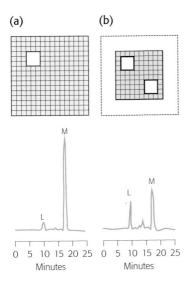

Figure 5.3 The intestinal permeability test. The monosaccharide crosses the mucosa through water filled intracellular pores (small squares), while the disaccharide is larger and can permeate only through the intercellular junctions (large squares). (a) Normal mucosa and its high performance liquid chromatography (HPLC) pattern of urinary recovery of permeability probes. (b) When the mucosa is damaged the number of water-filled pores decreases due to a reduction in absorptive surface, while intercellular permeation increases. This is reflected by a decreased recovery of mannitol and increased recovery of lactulose in the urine. M, mannitol; L, lactulose.

43

surface) is usually found. It should be noted, however, that the results can be normal in some patients with either atypical or silent coeliac disease, probably because the mucosal damage extends only a short way down the bowel. In practice, the permeability test offers no advantages over serological tests.

Imaging

Bowel radiology. Dilatation of the small bowel with thickening of the mucosal folds and clumping of the barium are features seen on follow-through examination (Figure 5.4). It is not necessary to perform such investigations routinely, but they should be considered if:

- patients are unusually ill at presentation with dramatic weight loss, abdominal pain, features of intestinal obstruction or have abdominal masses
- blood tests show marked abnormalities (e.g. severe anaemia, low albumin)
- occult blood loss is found
- newly diagnosed patients do not show the expected responses to a GFD or response is lost in established cases.

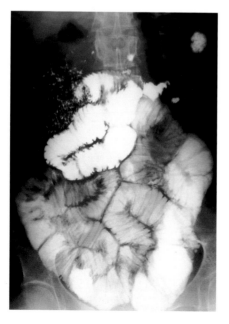

Figure 5.4 The appearance of the small bowel in untreated coeliac disease on barium follow-through examination, showing dilatation of the bowel and coarsening of the valvulae.

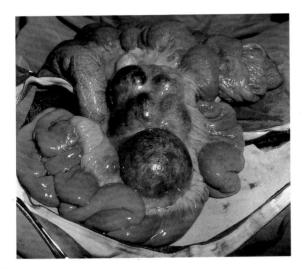

Figure 5.5 Mesentery of the small bowel in a patient with coeliac disease showing large cavitating lymph nodes.

Under these circumstances, a small bowel lymphoma or carcinoma, or jejunoileitis may be present.

Scanning. Ultrasound, computerized tomography (CT) and magnetic resonance imaging (MRI) may be helpful in patients who are severely ill at presentation, who do not show the expected responses to gluten withdrawal and in those in whom the response is lost. Enlarged lymph nodes denoting lymphoma or mesenteric lymph node cavitation syndrome may be found (Figure 5.5).

CHAPTER 6

Complications

Patients with coeliac disease, particularly those who are undiagnosed or do not adhere to a strict GFD, are prone to develop complications. Malignant complications are the most serious and should be suspected when expected responses to GFD are not achieved or sustained. Non-malignant complications can, however, also be troublesome and even life-threatening. Prevention is better than cure and it is important that patients are diagnosed before complications occur, because a GFD may prevent or reduce the risks of these developing.

Malignant complications

Lymphoma and other malignant tumours, particularly carcinoma of the oesophagus and jejunum, are associated with coeliac disease.

Aetiology. The aetiology of malignant complications is unknown, but local and general mechanisms have to be considered.
- The mucosal lesion is premalignant.
- Carcinogens may penetrate the abnormally permeable mucosa.
- The mucosa may be deficient in carcinogen-detoxifying enzymes.
- Abnormalities in the immune system may predispose to tumour formation.
- Immune disturbances may allow oncogenic viruses to replicate.
- The HLA status may predispose to malignancy.

Prevalence. The prevalence of malignant complications is unknown for several reasons.
- The prevalence of coeliac disease in the population is unknown, because many patients without symptoms or only mild complaints may never be diagnosed.
- If autopsies are not performed, the presence of malignancy will be underestimated.
- Patients with lymphoma or other malignancy may have coeliac disease that remains undiagnosed.

- Data reported from referral centres are unlikely to reflect the fate of coeliac patients in the general population.
- The wider use of a GFD is altering the risk of developing lymphoma.
- Some coeliac populations may be at greater risk than others.

Nevertheless, data from groups of patients followed up for many years show that the prevalence of gastrointestinal cancers is 3–11% and lymphoma 0–7%.

From a carefully documented series of 262 coeliac patients diagnosed over 26 years (1972–97) in Derby, UK, calculations indicate that, in patients with coeliac disease, 60 lymphomas may occur each year in the UK. However, these results may not apply to other localities. It must also be emphasized that these results apply only to a defined coeliac population and may not be true for all coeliac patients.

Lymphoma is of T-cell origin and is now referred to as enteropathy-associated T-cell lymphoma (EATL). This type of lymphoma can occur in the absence of enteropathy, suggesting that EATL is a clinical rather than pathological entity. A monoclonal antibody HML-1, developed against IEL, also stains these lymphoma cells. In coeliac disease, there is an expansion of the $CD3^+,CD7^+, CD4^-, CD8^-$ IEL population and the phenotype of EATL suggests an origin from these double-negative cells.

Clinical presentation. Lymphoma in patients with coeliac disease presents in one of two ways.

- The diagnosis of coeliac disease clearly precedes the onset of symptoms attributed to malignancy. These patients have responded to a GFD then deteriorate because of the onset of lymphoma.
- Coeliac disease and lymphoma present together, or within a short interval of time. Whether these patients have coeliac disease has been the subject of controversy. However, evidence indicates that the development of lymphoma is the event that brings coeliac disease to attention. When compared with uncomplicated patients with coeliac disease, this group has a similar HLA profile, similar changes in intraepithelial subsets, and a similar incidence of hyposplenism. Furthermore, the presence of the genotype associated with coeliac disease, DQA1*0501, DQB1*0201, and immunohistochemical studies of EATL also support this view.

Weight loss, lethargy, diarrhoea, abdominal pain, muscle weakness, finger-clubbing, pyrexia and lymphadenopathy are symptoms that point to the diagnosis of lymphoma. In most patients the illness is insidious, but presentation can be acute with intestinal perforation, obstruction or bleeding from the tumour (Figures 6.1 and 6.2).

Diagnosis. The diagnosis of lymphoma can be difficult and delayed because the presenting features are often non-specific and similar to those encountered in coeliac disease at diagnosis or in relapse. In about one-third of cases, the diagnosis is made only at autopsy.

Many haematological and biochemical abnormalities occur in coeliac patients with lymphoma, but no pattern that allows early diagnosis has been found. A progressive rise in serum IgA is sometimes seen, but this may also

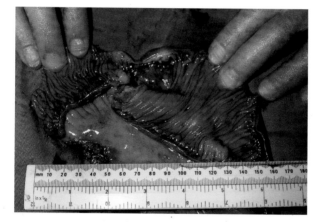

Figure 6.1
Obstructing lymphoma in the jejunum.

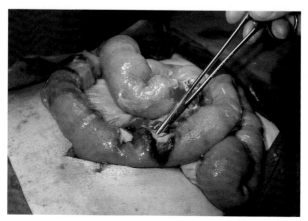

Figure 6.2
Multifocal small intestinal lymphoma with perforation.

occur in coeliac disease without malignancy. Increased levels of serum lysozyme occur, but are not a reliable indicator of lymphoma. Lower plasma cell and higher lymphocyte counts in the lamina propria and lower lymphocyte counts in the epithelium have been reported in small bowel biopsies from patients who eventually develop lymphoma compared with those who do not. Hypoplastic crypts and histiocytic aggregates have also been reported. Unfortunately, these observations are not helpful in individual patients.

Bowel radiography is essential if lymphoma is suspected and will reveal multiple, irregular, narrowed segments characteristic of small bowel involvement (Figure 6.3). Lesions may, however, not be seen on radiography and only a malabsorption pattern seen. Upper gastrointestinal endoscopy, which is now the preferred method for diagnosing coeliac disease, allows inspection of the oesophagus, stomach and proximal duodenum. Enteroscopy enables more of the small bowel to be visualized, but intestinal perforation is a risk and the technique is still being evaluated. Enteroscopy with mucosal biopsy will reveal jejunoileitis, which is also a cause of deterioration in coeliac disease and may be associated with lymphoma (see page 50). The roles of ultrasound, CT and MRI are still to be determined; these techniques will detect mesenteric lymph node cavitation, which may be mistaken clinically for lymphoma (see Figure 5.5). Laparotomy may be necessary when lymphoma is suspected, but a firm diagnosis has not been made. This can be a difficult decision in an ill patient and surgery may contribute to mortality. On the other hand, it is sometimes possible to perform a curative operation for a localized lesion.

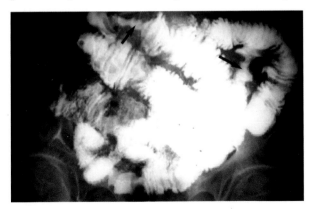

Figure 6.3
Barium study showing two lymphomatous strictures (arrowed) in the small bowel.

49

Pathology. Although most lymphomas are located in the jejunum, they may also be found in the ileum and lymph nodes, and less commonly in the stomach and colon. They occur as solitary or multiple circumferential ulcerating lesions, mucosal plaques or nodules. The histological appearance is variable, but the tumours are of high grade and large cell type. The mucosa of adjacent bowel is flat.

Carcinoma. As for lymphoma, the development of carcinoma may bring a patient with coeliac disease to diagnosis or provoke symptoms in a patient previously well controlled on a GFD.

Carcinoma of oesophagus usually presents with dysphagia, anaemia or bleeding and can be diagnosed by biopsy at endoscopy.

Carcinoma of jejunum. Anaemia is the most common presenting feature and is often associated with either overt or occult gastrointestinal blood loss. Weight loss, abdominal pain and intestinal obstruction are other prominent complaints. If the tumour is in the proximal duodenum, it may be visualized at endoscopy. Barium studies will usually detect lesions further down the intestine or show evidence of obstruction.

Other groups at risk

Dermatitis herpetiformis. Patients with dermatitis herpetiformis have a higher than normal risk of developing lymphoma (up to 2.8%), but may not be at increased risk of carcinoma of the gastrointestinal tract.

Relatives of patients with coeliac disease. No increase in lymphoma has been observed, but a higher risk of oesophageal cancer has been found in the only study to address this issue.

Ulcerative jejunoileitis is an uncommon complication of coeliac disease in which chronic ulcers are found mainly in the jejunum and ileum (see page 55). It can be difficult to differentiate from bowel lymphoma clinically and radiologically. In addition, both disorders may occur together in the same patient and sometimes ulceration will be diagnosed before lymphoma becomes apparent.

Treatment and prognosis. Surgery, radiotherapy and chemotherapy may be used in suitable cases depending on the site of lesions and staging. If tumours are confined to the gastrointestinal tract, resection of the affected segment (or segments) may result in cure. In most patients, lymphoma is widespread at diagnosis and the outlook is poor, although may be improving with chemotherapy and surgery. Survival at 1 year and at 5 years may be 30% and 10%, respectively.

Effect of gluten-free diet on malignancy. Because of the difficulties in making an early diagnosis of lymphoma and the poor prognosis, attention has turned to prevention and the role that a GFD might play. A GFD restores the structure and function of the small bowel towards normal and might, therefore, reduce the malignant potential.

A study investigating the effect of a GFD on the risk of malignancy has been carried out in Birmingham, UK. Of the 210 patients, 108 followed a strict GFD, while the remainder had a normal or reduced gluten diet. In the group that had taken a strict GFD for 5 or more consecutive years, the overall risk of malignancy was not significantly increased compared with that of the general population. For those ingesting gluten, however, the risk was significantly increased. Excess morbidity was also calculated and was clearly related to the amount of gluten ingested (Table 6.1).

TABLE 6.1

Effect of diet on morbidity in cancer of the mouth, pharynx and oesophagus, and lymphoma in patients with coeliac disease

Diet	Number of patients	Morbidity rate				Excess morbidity rate*
		Observed	Expected	Observed/ expected	p value	
Normal	46	7	0.19	36.8	<0.001	10.7
Reduced gluten	56	5	0.12	41.7	<0.001	5.0
Strict gluten free	108	3	0.46	6.5	<0.05	1.2

*Excess morbidity rate = $\dfrac{\text{Observed} - \text{expected}}{\text{Person years at risk} \times 10^3}$

Trend for excess morbidity rate over diet group: $\chi^2_1 = 9.9$; $p < 0.01$.

Study of lymphoma in dermatitis herpetiformis has also shown a GFD to be protective. These results indicate that a GFD does reduce the malignant risk and is a further reason to advise all patients to adhere to a strict diet for life.

Approach to patients. Patients are becoming increasingly aware of the link between coeliac disease and malignancy, and would like further information. This is a very sensitive area and a thoughtful approach is required so that patients do not become unduly alarmed. It is now possible to adopt an encouraging and positive attitude, and advise patients that the best insurance against the development of malignant complications is strict adherence to a GFD for life.

Non-malignant complications

Disorders of bone and calcium metabolism. Coeliac disease predisposes to abnormalities of bone and calcium metabolism, which result in rickets, osteomalacia and osteoporosis. The introduction of modern techniques that allow the accurate measurement of bone mineral density, parathyroid hormone concentrations, vitamin D metabolites, and markers of bone formation and resorption have provided new means of exploring these facets of coeliac disease.

Pathogenesis. The pathogenesis of osteopenia is not fully understood, but the development of hypocalcaemia is likely to be the central event that leads to parathyroid hormone release and bone resorption. A number of mechanisms lead to hypocalcaemia:

- a reduced intake of calcium
- associated lactose intolerance restricting milk and therefore calcium intake
- increased endogenous loss
- loss of surface area for absorption
- low concentration of 25-hydroxycholecalciferol
- reduced responsiveness of the small bowel to 1,25-dihydroxy-cholecalciferol promoting malabsorption of calcium
- reduction of calcium transport proteins (e.g. calbindin).

Increased concentrations of 1,25-dihydroxycholecalciferol are found in patients taking a normal diet because the enzyme 1-α-hydroxylase is enhanced. The levels fall in those taking a GFD, but may remain above normal, possibly accounting for the incomplete recovery of bone mass observed in some treated patients. A GFD also tends to normalize parathyroid hormone and serum calcium. The markers of bone remodelling, osteocalcin and serum carboxy-terminal propeptide of type 1 procollagen (markers of formation), and serum carboxy-terminal pyridinolone cross-linked telopeptide of type 1 collagen (a marker of resorption), are significantly increased in untreated compared with treated patients and indicate increased bone turnover.

Clinical features and diagnosis. The severe clinical forms of osteomalacia are now rarely seen and the present challenge is to detect those patients who have none or only minor symptoms of coeliac or bone disease. Early recognition and treatment will prevent more severe problems arising. Osteomalacia can occur in the absence of gastrointestinal symptoms or steatorrhoea, and may be the presenting complaint. Myopathy may be a prominent presenting feature of osteomalacia in coeliac patients.

Biochemical profiles that are routine in most hospitals, including calcium, phosphate and alkaline phosphatase, may indicate the presence of osteomalacia. Further investigations, such as assay of vitamin D metabolites and bone biopsy may be undertaken, but are not usually necessary. Monitoring the response to a GFD and vitamin D by symptoms, if present, and changes in the blood chemistry may be sufficient.

Treatment. The aim of treatment is to restore the small intestinal mucosa to normal by adopting a GFD, so that the mechanisms which promote calcium absorption can become fully effective. Improvements in bone scores can be detected within 1 year of beginning a GFD and the bones may return to normal after 4–10 years. In children and adolescents, a GFD alone can restore bone density, but in adults, other treatments such as calcium supplements, vitamin D, hormone replacement and bisphosphonates may be required.

Splenic atrophy and hyposplenism. Hyposplenism with or without splenic atrophy can affect up to 75% of adult patients, but is not seen in children. Assessed by pitted red cell counts, a GFD improves hyposplenism in some patients. In most patients, hyposplenism is not detrimental and does not predispose to malignancy, but can occasionally be associated with overwhelming infection. Infection in coeliac patients, particularly those who are debilitated, should be treated quickly and administration of pneumococcal vaccine should be considered.

Neurological and psychiatric disorders. The prevalence of neurological and psychiatric disorders in coeliac disease is unknown and most are encountered as single cases, even in large clinics. Which disorders, if any, are specific for coeliac disease is also unknown. Patients most commonly present with ataxia due to cerebellar or spinocerebellar degeneration or with features of peripheral neuropathy. Epilepsy is more common in coeliac patients, occurring in 3–5%. There is an association between coeliac disease, epilepsy and intracranial calcifications (Figure 6.4), though why these phenomena should be present together is not understood. The geographical distribution of these latter patients is also puzzling, as most have occurred in Italy and none, so far, in the UK. Depression affects about 10% of coeliac patients on a normal diet and, in some cases, is severe and leads to suicide.

Whether these disorders arise as a result of deficiencies due to malabsorption or because of an underlying mechanism inherent in coeliac disease, possibly related to gluten, is unknown. Some patients with peripheral neuropathy may improve when given a GFD and vitamin supplements. A GFD may reduce or halt seizures in some patients with epilepsy. There is no treatment for the severe neuropathies that affect the central nervous system.

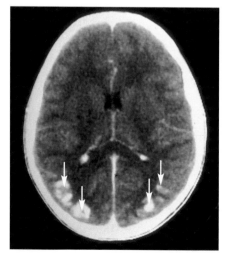

Figure 6.4 MRI scan showing intracranial calcifications in a patient with coeliac disease and epilepsy.

Reproductive disorders

Menarche and menopause. Menarche is late and the menopause early in untreated coeliac patients compared with those who are treated and controls, so that the reproductive period is reduced for those on normal diet.

Infertility and pregnancy. Coeliac disease is a cause of infertility, but if bowel symptoms are mild or absent, the diagnosis may be missed. Giving a GFD or folic acid may result in conception. Men with coeliac disease may have reversible infertility. Impotence, hypogonadism, and abnormal sperm motility and forms occur. Recurrent abortion is a feature of untreated coeliac disease and successful pregnancy may ensue after gluten withdrawal.

Ulcerative jejunoileitis is characterized by malabsorption, almost always a flat small intestinal biopsy and chronic ulcers found mainly in the jejunum and ileum, but rarely in the colon (Figure 6.5). It is likely that most patients have underlying coeliac disease. The development of jejunoileitis may bring a patient with coeliac disease to diagnosis or cause deterioration in those previously well controlled on a GFD, as may occur with malignancy. It may be premalignant or even a low-grade malignant condition from the onset.

Symptoms and signs include fever, anorexia, weight loss, dehydration, oedema, diarrhoea and abdominal pain. Patients with suspected ulcerative jejunoileitis should be admitted to hospital, because deterioration is usually relentless and rapid. Initial treatment consists of rehydration with correction of electrolyte disturbances. Intravenous steroids should be given from the

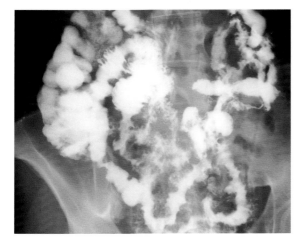

Figure 6.5 Ulcerative jejunoileitis. The small bowel shows a very abnormal pattern with ulceration, thickening of the wall and narrowing of the lumen.

outset. Anaemia often requires blood transfusion and deficiencies of folic acid, ferritin and vitamins B_{12}, D and K need to be corrected. Malnutrition and hypoalbuminaemia are usually marked and require prolonged parenteral feeding. Azathioprine is useful for those not controlled by steroids or needing large doses. Improvement is measured by weight gain and increases in serum albumin concentration. For those who present with intestinal perforation, obstruction or bleeding from the bowel, urgent surgery will be necessary. When enteral feeding becomes possible, a GFD should be given. Milk restriction in the early months may improve symptoms of abdominal bloating, wind and diarrhoea. This is a serious complication with a high mortality, but with intensive support full recovery is possible.

Mesenteric lymph node cavitation is a rare, serious complication that affects those with long-standing, untreated coeliac disease and should also be suspected in patients who are not responding to a GFD (see Figure 5.5). The condition may be more common than currently thought and it is likely that the increasing use of ultrasound and CT scanning will bring more cases to light. Abdominal masses due to enlarged, cystic lymph nodes may be confused with malignant tumours so that an accurate diagnosis is essential. The prognosis is grave, but recovery is possible. Supportive treatments as for ulcerative jejunoileitis are given.

CHAPTER 7

Management

The treatment of coeliac disease is based on the lifelong exclusion of gluten-containing cereals from the diet. In many areas of the world, including Europe, North America, Australasia and North Africa, gluten-rich products, such as bread and pasta, are part of the staple diet. Gluten-containing foods therefore make a substantial contribution to daily energy intake and are enjoyable to eat. The changes needed to begin and maintain a GFD are substantial and have a major impact on daily life. Thus, starting the diet is a critical step that should be handled sympathetically by experienced doctors and dietitians. The rationale for and the benefits of the diet require careful explanation, placing emphasis on the wide range of foods that can be eaten rather than just on those that have to be excluded.

The gluten-free diet

Wheat, barley and rye derivatives are excluded in the GFD. Although the toxicity of oats has recently been questioned, as ingestion has not caused any histological or clinical deterioration in either patients with coeliac disease or dermatitis herpetiformis, the long-term consequences are still unclear and it remains the current practice to exclude them from the diet. Spelt is an inferior species of wheat grown in the mountainous parts of Europe and must also be excluded. Cereals that do not contain gluten and can be eaten include rice and maize. Other natural foods, such as vegetables, salads, pulses, buckwheat, fruits, nuts, meat, fish, poultry, cheese, eggs and milk, can also be eaten without limitation. A wide range of attractive and palatable gluten-free products that guarantee the absence of gluten are specifically manufactured for coeliac patients and may be labelled by an internationally recognized mark, the crossed ear of wheat. There are difficulties, however, in maintaining a strict GFD diet because of 'hidden gluten', inadequate food labelling and food contamination.

Hidden gluten. Many commercial products, ready meals and convenience foods are made with wheat flour, gluten-containing wheat proteins or gluten-containing starches added as a filler, stabilizing agent or processing aid. These include sausages, fish fingers, cheese spreads, soups, sauces, mixed seasonings, mincemeat for mince pies, and some medications and vitamin preparations. All real ales, beers, lagers and stout should be avoided, but spirits, wines, liqueurs and ciders are allowed. Whisky and malt whisky are allowed.

National coeliac societies in many countries publish handbooks that list the gluten-free products which are available. These handbooks are regularly updated and are essential for coeliac patients to have in their possession. It is important to remember that food lists are only applicable for use in the country in which they were compiled. Similar foods with well-known brand names may be made under franchise in different countries to slightly different recipes; they may look and taste the same, but be gluten free in one country and not in others.

Food labelling. Coeliac patients are only able to decide what products are unsuitable for them by reading food labels. Some foods may, unknown to patients because of imprecise labelling, contain gluten and be eaten. Coeliac societies, in many cases, will have ascertained from food manufacturers which products are safe and these will be included in the food lists. There are still pitfalls, however, when information is unavailable, and products containing starch and modified starch should only be taken when its origin is known.

Food labelling directives must be improved in the Codex Standards, in the EU and nationally. The Codex Alimentarius Commission, a joint venture of the Food and Agriculture Organization of the United Nations and the World Health Organization, elaborates Codex Standards for food labelling through committees in a complex process of negotiation. Codex Standards are usually adopted by national governments. At present, about 160 governments representing 97% of the world population are members of the Commission. In addition, over 100 non-governmental organizations, including the Association of European Coeliac Societies (AOECS), are accepted as observers. Lobbying by AOECS has influenced the Commission and the EU on labelling directives. For example, by the year 2001, food labels in the EU will have to show the specific vegetable origin of starches and modified starches if they contain gluten.

Contamination. Grains that are naturally gluten free can become contaminated with wheat, particularly when the same mills are used to process different cereals. Similarly, gluten-free products may be contaminated when they are produced using the same production lines and equipment employed for making gluten-containing foods. These problems are difficult to overcome, but some companies are beginning to use dedicated production lines.

Recently, research into the use of gluten to coat foods such as fruits, vegetables and cheeses to preserve moisture and flavour was initiated. Under pressure from AOECS, the tests were stopped – foods that are naturally gluten free must remain uncontaminated and therefore safe for coeliac patients to consume.

Compliance with the gluten-free diet

Studies have shown that between 45% and 94% of patients adhere to a strict GFD. This wide variation reflects, to some extent, whether the study population was made up of children or adults, the proportion with few or no symptoms, and the closeness of follow up. Strict dietary compliance is a problem for a number of reasons.

- A GFD imposes restrictions on everyday lifestyle.
- Maintaining a GFD when travelling, eating out, dining with friends and on holiday can be particularly difficult.
- Adolescents may break the diet because of peer pressure and a sense of not wanting to be different from their friends. During this period of life, gluten can be ingested without producing symptoms, which is another reason for non-compliance at this time.
- Patients with silent coeliac disease (i.e. a flat biopsy but no symptoms) have little incentive to adhere strictly to the diet because they regard themselves as well.
- A GFD is more expensive than a normal diet.

Serological tests to monitor dietary compliance. After a GFD has been initiated, IgA AGA reduces to normal within a few months and this value can be used as an index of dietary compliance (Figure 5.1, page 40). Abnormal IgG AGA levels may persist longer due to so-called immunological memory. IgA AEA also disappears in those on a strict GFD.

It should be noted that AGA and AEA are too insensitive to detect minor transgressions of the diet.

Risk associated with ingesting small amounts of gluten

Quite apart from non-compliance, gluten may be present in an apparently GFD for the reasons outlined above. Patients often ask whether eating small amounts of gluten regularly or occasionally will be harmful. The best advice is that they should adhere strictly to the diet, but it has to be conceded that the risks associated with the protracted ingestion of very small amounts of gluten are still unclear. Although most patients will not experience any

(a)

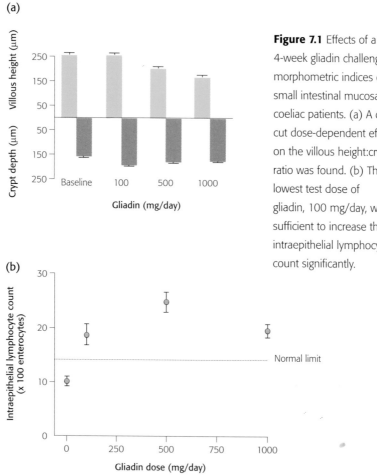

Figure 7.1 Effects of a 4-week gliadin challenge on morphometric indices of the small intestinal mucosa in coeliac patients. (a) A clear-cut dose-dependent effect on the villous height:crypt ratio was found. (b) The lowest test dose of gliadin, 100 mg/day, was sufficient to increase the intraepithelial lymphocyte count significantly.

clinical symptoms if they eat small amounts of gluten, it has been shown that deterioration of the intestinal mucosal architecture may ensue with increased IEL counts, which is the most sensitive index to detect abnormalities (Figure 7.1). It should be noted that in some countries, including the UK, the GFD is based on wheat starch and this can contain gluten up to 200 ppm (20 mg/100 g). This product has served patients well for 50 years and many studies demonstrating the benefits of gluten withdrawal, including reducing the lymphoma risk, have employed this diet.

Other treatments

While virtually all children respond well to a GFD, 10–15% of adult patients do not and additional measures have to be employed.

Restriction of dairy products. In untreated coeliac disease, the small intestinal enterocytes are severely damaged resulting in disaccharidase deficiency. This may cause persistent diarrhoea and abdominal bloating if milk and dairy products are ingested. As the morphology of the mucosa improves, lactase activity tends to return to normal within a few months. In some cases, avoidance or reduction of lactose-containing products may be indicated for a short period after diagnosis before full-strength cows' milk and dairy products can be reintroduced in the diet. A few patients can never tolerate these foods and have to exclude them for life. Under these circumstances, dietary calcium intake will be reduced and it is wise to give supplements.

Restriction of other foods. Rarely, some patients only return to full health when foods such as eggs, chicken, tuna and soy are removed from the diet. Great care needs to be taken not to exclude foods to which patients may not in fact be sensitive. Restriction of dairy products and other foods must be carefully monitored, because as the diet becomes more limited, compliance is often jeopardized.

Steroids. A few adult patients are severely ill at presentation and may benefit from a short course of steroids while the GFD is taking effect. Some may require a small dose of steroids over a prolonged period to keep them in good health. Children never require steroids in this way.

Supplements. Patients are often deficient in iron, folic acid, calcium and vitamin D, and supplements should be given as required.

Response to treatment

After starting a GFD, symptomatic children show progressive clinical improvement and weight gain that parallel the healing of the coeliac enteropathy. The first signs of amelioration are often seen within a few days, with increased appetite and mood change, but it may take some months before symptoms disappear completely. In typical cases, the response to treatment is sometimes prodigious, so that a severely malnourished and miserable child is rapidly transformed into a sturdy and healthy youngster.

Most adults also respond dramatically to a GFD, and the clinical and morphological improvements usually occur in parallel, though clinical improvement can occur without improvement in the biopsy appearances.

Follow up

Patients should be followed up for life, preferably in a specialist clinic, otherwise they are more likely to stray from the GFD. Those taking gluten, either accidentally or on purpose, may well suffer ill health and be exposed to health risks including malignancy and osteoporosis. After diagnosis and the introduction of a GFD, patients should be reviewed at about 3 months and again at 6 months to ensure that they are making satisfactory progress and managing the diet. If all is well, they should be reviewed annually, or sooner if problems arise. This is advisable in order that:

- any health concerns and associated disorders or complications that may have arisen can be addressed
- weight in adults, and growth and development in children, can be monitored
- blood tests can be carried out to monitor haematological and biochemical indices, particularly haemoglobin, iron, folate and calcium
- adherence to the GFD can be assessed by dietary history and measurement of AGA and AEA
- the need for other investigations, such as further small bowel biopsies and scans for osteoporosis, can be assessed
- current membership of a Coeliac Society is confirmed.

Advice for coeliac families

Parents with coeliac disease, or other relatives with the condition, often ask whether their children are likely to develop the disorder. Coeliac disease does run in families, but not in a predictable fashion. If the disorder is present in a family, the chance of another member being affected is about 1 in 10. Family members can now be screened easily with serological tests and small intestinal biopsies should be carried out in those who are positive.

When a new baby is born into a family with coeliac disease, parents should be advised to introduce gluten at the same age as for any child. All babies are usually now weaned on gluten-free foods and wheat cereals are not introduced until 6–9 months of age. After this period, normal gluten intake should be achieved. It is important that babies are fed normally rather than given a GFD, so that if coeliac disease is present, it will become evident, and can be diagnosed and treated promptly.

Role of coeliac societies

At the time of diagnosis, all coeliac patients should be advised to join their National Coeliac Society and support one of the local groups in their area. These non-profit-making organizations, which are made up of and run by coeliac patients and their families, fulfil a number of important functions by:

- helping patients to follow the GFD by producing comprehensive handbooks of the gluten-free foods that are available
- acting as a stimulus so that companies produce a wide range of palatable, attractive foods
- encouraging hotels and restaurants to cater for coeliac patients
- promoting meetings and producing videos, journals and other literature designed to inform patients about the condition
- raising the profile of coeliac disease in the community
- raising funds for research into coeliac disease.

CHAPTER 8

Dermatitis herpetiformis

Dermatitis herpetiformis (DH) was named by Duhring in 1884, although his original description covered several disorders and included conditions such as pemphigoid, pemphigus, herpes gestationis and erythema multiforme. With the development of histological and immunofluorescence techniques and treatments, DH was subsequently shown to be a specific disorder. In 1940, it was observed that the rash was suppressed by sulphapyridine, and 10 years later, dapsone was found to be even more effective. In the 1960s, two important developments occurred. An enteropathy was found in patients with DH, similar to that found in coeliac disease, and IgA deposits were detected in apparently normal skin, which formed the basis of a diagnostic test.

Epidemiology

DH occurs most commonly in individuals of European origin. The prevalence is approximately 10/100 000 in the UK, although higher rates of 40/100 000 and 66/100 000 have been reported from centres in Sweden and Finland, respectively. DH seldom occurs in Asians and, like coeliac disease, is unknown in blacks. DH can present at any age, but is rare at the extremes of life; the mean age at presentation is about 40 years. In contrast with coeliac disease, for which the male to female patient ratio is 1:1.3, DH is more common in men than women (1.5–1.9:1).

Family studies indicate that 5% of first-degree relatives will also have DH and 5% coeliac disease; the relatives of patients with these conditions should always be screened. Both conditions are associated with the class II HLA DQw2 molecule and particularly with the heterodimer DQα1*0501, DQβ1*0201. Monozygotic twins, of whom one has DH and the other coeliac disease, are known. These observations emphasize the link between the two disorders.

Aetiology

It is not known why only some patients with coeliac disease develop DH and what factors link the bowel and skin lesions. In DH, IgA is present in the skin, inflammatory cells and cytokines are found in the lesions, AGA and anti-connective tissue antibodies (e.g. ARA, AEA) occur in the serum and gastrointestinal secretions, and the rash is gluten sensitive. The importance of these factors and how they interact to produce skin lesions remains unknown.

An early hypothesis proposed that gluten–antigluten immune complexes were central in the pathogenesis of DH and, by binding to reticulin in the skin, produced the lesions. Gluten, however, has never been found in skin lesions, although it may be present in a form that is difficult to detect. IgA is present in uninvolved skin, and is still present when the rash goes into remission, either spontaneously or following treatment. It is difficult to quantify IgA in the skin and, even on a strict GFD, it can take several years for this to clear from the skin.

Clinical features

Rash. The earliest abnormality consists of a small erythematous macule 2–3 mm in diameter, which rapidly develops into an urticarial papule. Small vesicles appear, which may coalesce and with scratching rupture, dry and form scabs. The vesicles are tense, shiny and filled with clear fluid, which clouds as the lesion progresses. Pustules are rare. Blisters take 7–10 days to involute and, at any one time, all stages of development will be present.

The predominant symptoms are intense itching and burning. Rupture of the blisters by scratching leads to rapid relief of symptoms and only evidence of excoriation may be seen at presentation. Healing is often complete, but areas of pigmentation and occasionally scars may remain. The rash has a characteristic symmetrical distribution and can be found on any part of the body except the soles of the feet. The elbows and upper forearms are affected in over 90% of patients (Figure 8.1). Other sites commonly involved are the buttocks, knees, shoulders, sacrum, face, scalp, neck and trunk. Oral lesions are found in 5% of cases. The rash may be widespread, but can be limited to one or two sites. Local trauma caused by, for example, belts, braces and straps, may precipitate lesions and, following inadequate drug treatment, the rash tends to reappear at the same sites.

Once the rash appears, it is a continuous problem in most patients, but it can run an intermittent course in 10% of cases. Lesions may be worse premenstrually, although pregnancy has a variable effect. DH tends to be less severe in the elderly and may be more likely to remit spontaneously. For

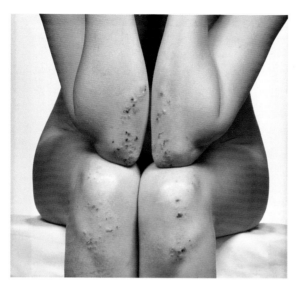

Figure 8.1 Blisters on the elbows and knees of a patient with dermatitis herpetiformis. Reproduced courtesy of T Reunala, Tampere, Finland.

those taking a normal diet, the spontaneous remission rate is around 10%, but the diagnosis in these atypical patients should be reviewed.

Associated enteropathy. Over 90% of patients with DH have no gastrointestinal symptoms. This may be because the mucosal abnormalities extend only a short distance into the small intestine with sufficient normal bowel to compensate. A few patients do, however, complain of diarrhoea or abdominal bloating, but severe symptoms are rare.

Villous atrophy in the upper small intestinal mucosa is found in 65–75% of patients with DH. Lesions are often patchy, and taking multiple biopsies using a fibre-optic endoscope increases the likelihood of detecting abnormalities. Even in patients with apparently normal biopsies, subtle changes in the mucosa, such as raised numbers of IEL and γ/δ T cells in the epithelium, alterations in intestinal humoral immunity and the production of villous atrophy with gluten challenge, indicate that all patients are gluten sensitive.

Associated endocrine and connective tissue disorders. DH is associated with endocrine or connective tissue disorders in about 5% of patients, and these problems usually develop prior to the diagnosis of DH. The most common endocrine problems are autoimmune thyroid disease and type 1 diabetes mellitus, and the connective tissue disorders include Sjögren's syndrome, lupus erythematosus, rheumatoid arthritis and scleroderma. It is important that these associated conditions are not overlooked at diagnosis of DH or during follow up.

Malignancy. Lymphoma or other types of malignancy may complicate DH and occur before, coincidentally, or after the diagnosis of DH is established.

Prognosis. The prognosis is good unless lymphoma develops, but this is unusual. It should be possible to control the rash with drugs and a GFD, although relapses may occur for no apparent reason from time to time.

Investigations

Histological findings in the skin are non-specific and take the form of papillary microabscesses and subepidermal blisters with a neutrophil infiltration. A 4-mm punch biopsy should be taken and snap frozen in liquid nitrogen for immunofluorescence studies, which can detect IgA deposits in the skin.

IgA deposits in skin. The diagnosis of DH rests on the demonstration of IgA in uninvolved skin. The most common site is in the dermal papillae, where IgA is detected as granular or fibrillar deposits (Figure 8.2). IgA may also be laid down in a linear granular fashion along the line of the basement membrane. It is important that this pattern is differentiated from homogeneous linear IgA deposition found in linear IgA disease, which is not gluten dependent. It has been claimed that if multiple sections of skin of one or two biopsies are carefully examined by a skilled observer, all patients with DH will show IgA deposits. The corollary of this is that the diagnosis of DH should not be accepted in the absence of these abnormalities.

Small bowel biopsy. A biopsy of the upper small bowel is required in all patients. These are usually obtained from the duodenum using standard fibre-optic endoscopes, which allow several specimens to be taken. If the biopsy appears to be normal or near normal by routine histology, more sophisticated tests will indicate subtle changes indicating gluten sensitivity as outlined above.

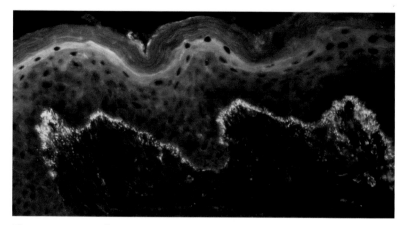

Figure 8.2 Immunofluorescence biopsy showing granular IgA deposits in the upper papillary dermis in a patient with dermatitis herpetiformis. Reproduced courtesy of T Reunala, Tampere, Finland.

Tests of malabsorption. Although patients may not have overt evidence of malabsorption, haemoglobin, ferritin, folate and B_{12} concentrations should be measured because deficiencies may exist. A reduced serum calcium and elevated alkaline phosphatase will indicate osteomalacia.

Imaging is required only if sinister symptoms, such as those suggestive of small bowel lymphoma, are present. In such cases, a barium follow-through study of the small bowel is required.

Differential diagnosis

While DH can be easily recognized in most cases because of its characteristic presentation, appearance and distribution, other disorders have to be considered in less typical cases. Difficulties arise when lesions are sparse and scratching has left only excoriations and scabs. In addition, rashes in some other conditions may appear clinically similar to DH and respond to sulphones. Disorders that have to be differentiated include eczema, linear IgA disease (LAD), pemphigoid and pemphigus.

The distribution of eczema differs from that of DH and is not confined to extensor surfaces. The lesions respond to topical and systemic steroids, and tests for immunofluorescence are negative. In some patients, dapsone will reduce the itch, which may cause confusion.

The blisters in LAD are similar to those seen in DH, but are not confined to extensor surfaces. A skin biopsy will show IgA deposited characteristically in a linear fashion along the dermato-epidermal junction. LAD of childhood also shows this staining pattern and the rash responds to dapsone.

Pemphigoid occurs in an older population and the tense blisters vary in size from a few millimetres to a few centimetres. The groin, axillae, flexures of the limbs and lower abdomen are most commonly involved. IgG is found at the dermato-epidermal junction. The disorder responds to steroids and, after treatment for 2–3 years, many patients remain in remission.

Pemphigus is characterized by thin-walled blisters, which are present in the mouth in 50% of cases. The intraepithelial blisters rupture easily to leave eroded areas prone to secondary infection. If lesions are extensive, fluid loss can lead to severe metabolic changes and death. Intercellular IgG is present in the skin. Steroids have improved the prognosis, but may contribute to mortality because of side-effects.

Treatment

The rash of DH responds rapidly to drug treatment, which is required by almost all patients because of severe irritation. A GFD should be advised and enables most patients ultimately to stop or reduce the drug dose. Supplements should be given to patients with nutritional deficiencies (e.g. iron, folate).

Drug treatments. The three drugs commonly used to control the rash are dapsone, sulphapyridine and sulphamethoxypyridazine. Remission is induced within 24–48 hours and the rash clears within a week. These agents are so effective that if treatment fails, the diagnosis should be reviewed. Lesions return rapidly if the drugs are withdrawn before a GFD has had time to act.

Dapsone is the most widely used agent. Initially, it should be given in a dose of 100 mg, which is effective in most patients. Larger doses may be used, but are seldom required. It is not usually possible to reduce the dose until the patient has been on a GFD for about 6 months. Side-effects include anorexia, nausea, vomiting, insomnia, headache, neuropathy and hypoalbuminaemia. Haemolysis is common, as evidenced by a macrocytosis, and methaemoglobinaemia also occurs. Only rarely are these side-effects of clinical importance and an indication to change to another agent.

Sulphapyridine and sulphamethoxypyridazine may be used instead of, or in combination with, dapsone.

Gluten-free diet. All patients should be offered a GFD, even when the small intestinal mucosa appears normal, because the rash of DH is gluten sensitive. They should be interviewed by a dietitian and advised to adhere strictly to the diet. Patients may be reluctant to start or continue with a GFD, because only a few have gastrointestinal symptoms, which are usually mild. Following a GFD and with the benefit of hindsight, however, many patients do experience more energy and a greater sense of well-being. If it is carefully explained to them that this course of action may have a beneficial effect on their skin and avoid the necessity for long-term medication, they are much more likely to comply. Other benefits of a GFD include a reduction in malignant and non-malignant complications.

Whether patients can stop medication depends on their adherence to and time on a GFD. Of those patients who adhere strictly to a GFD, over 90% will be able to discontinue medication after 2 years. Less than 50% of those who continue to ingest some gluten are able to stop drug treatment, and the time to achieve this is 4–6 years. Those who elect to take a normal diet will require medication to suppress the rash unless they go into spontaneous remission.

CHAPTER 9

Future trends

In recent years, concepts of coeliac disease have undergone a revolution and have paved the way for further developments. With the advent of astonishingly sophisticated techniques in molecular medicine, advances in knowledge are assured and a new phase in the understanding of coeliac disease is dawning.

Mechanisms causing mucosal damage

The most favoured view is that mucosal damage is linked to the activation of T lymphocytes in the lamina propria by class II HLA-restricted gliadin-presenting cells. This triggers a cascade of reactions leading to and sustaining mucosal damage. T-cell reactions, however, do not appear to explain the whole pathogenesis and the influence of other cells, such as macrophages and their cytokines, will require detailed consideration. Whether non-immunological mechanisms also cause damage and why only some people become sensitized to gluten is unknown and research will continue to focus on these aspects. More detailed knowledge of the trimolecular complex of T-cell receptor, the major histocompatibility complex molecule and the damaging gliadin fragment will be forthcoming, and will help not only to explain aetiology and pathogenesis, but also to develop new approaches to treatment. The development of an animal model would greatly accelerate progress.

Diagnosis

Diagnosis still rests on finding a characteristic, severe enteropathy on histological examination of small bowel biopsies. It is, however, now clear that this is only one aspect of gluten sensitivity. Attention will focus on those patients with suspected coeliac disease whose small intestinal biopsies appear normal or near normal; such patients, in whom AEA can be detected in the serum and who have evidence of gluten sensitivity, have already been described. Diagnosis is important because a GFD restores health in those with symptoms and may prevent the future development of coeliac disease with a severe enteropathy and all the attendant health risks.

Why some patients with gluten sensitivity should have a normal biopsy, but others a severe enteropathy, is unknown. It may be that distinct genetic factors regulate susceptibility to gluten sensitivity and enteropathy. It appears that the form without severe enteropathy is less likely to be associated with the HLA alleles DQA1*0501, DQB1*0201, found in about 90% of those with classic coeliac disease.

In the near future, it is likely that serological and genetic markers will define coeliac disease more accurately and reduce the requirement for intestinal biopsy.

Treatments

While a GFD is a satisfactory treatment, patients often ask if a cure is on the horizon, by which they mean is it likely that they will ever be able to tolerate a normal diet? Researchers are addressing this issue but, clearly, alternative treatments must be safe and acceptable in the long term. An obvious solution would be to develop a strain of wheat that does not contain the toxic protein. Deleting the genes coding for α-gliadin in cultivar Chinese spring does not remove its damaging effects. This is not unexpected as it is likely that all gliadins cause tissue damage. If all gliadins were to be deleted, however, the resulting product might be safe, but would probably be no more palatable than the gluten-free breads that currently exist. Although this approach has so far been unrewarding, research continues because it is still possible that different wheats might have different tissue-damaging potential.

Another approach to treatment is to block, at some point, the cascade of immunological reactions that ultimately leads to tissue damage. This could be achieved at the level of T-cell activation or by modulating the effects of tissue-damaging agents that are produced.

The expression of experimental allergic encephalomyelitis in animals has been modified by blocking T-cell receptors using monoclonal antibodies or by vaccination with T-cell receptor peptides. Disruption of the CD28 co-stimulatory pathway has been used successfully in animals to modify immunological disorders and prolong graft survival. In tissue culture experiments, mucosal tolerance to gliadin can be induced by disturbing this same co-stimulatory activity. IFN-γ is produced in excess in the mucosa of patients with untreated coeliac disease and the consequent damage to the enterocytes can be prevented by anti-IFN-γ antibody. T cells exist in two subsets, Th1 and Th2, that produce a variety of cytokines. Th1 cells produce the damaging products IL-2 and IFN-γ, while Th2 cells are considered to protect against the development of autoimmune disease and produce the anti-inflammatory cytokines IL-4 and IL-10. In mice, induction of Th2 responses by giving antigen nasally has been shown to prevent murine type 1 diabetes mellitus. These observations offer the hope of developing new treatments for coeliac disease.

Awareness of coeliac disease

Coeliac disease is under-diagnosed. This is true not only for those with atypical presentations, but also for those with gastrointestinal complaints. This is unacceptable because there is a very effective treatment that not only restores patients to good health, but prevents complications. A greater awareness of the many ways that coeliac disease may present is essential. This will be achieved by wide dissemination of information through medical journals, in the undergraduate medical curriculum, in postgraduate meetings, by manufacturers of gluten-free foods and by coeliac societies. The increasing use of serological tests and endoscopic biopsy will uncover many more cases in the future.

The gluten-free diet

In recent years, the variety of gluten-free foods has increased enormously, mainly as a result of pressure from patients and their coeliac societies. Food labelling is, however, still unsatisfactory. Patients can be unaware that certain foods contain gluten because of imprecise information on food labels. There are moves to remedy some of the difficulties, but pressure in this area needs to be maintained.

Key references

GENERAL READING

Catassi C, Lifschitz CH, Giorgi PL, eds. Beyond the iceberg: The present and future of coeliac screening. *Acta Paediatrica* 1996;85(Suppl 412):1–84.

Howdle PD, ed. Coeliac disease. *Baillière's Clinical Gastroenterology.* Vol 9. London: Baillière Tindall, 1995.

Maki M, Collin P, Visakorpi JK. Coeliac disease. *Proceedings of the Seventh International Symposium on Coeliac Disease.* Tampere: Coeliac Disease Study Group, 1997.

Marsh MN, ed. *Coeliac Disease.* Oxford: Blackwell Scientific, 1992.

DEFINITION

Ferguson A, Arranz E, O'Mahony S. Clinical and pathological spectrum of coeliac disease. *Gut* 1993;34:150–1.

EPIDEMIOLOGY

Ascher H, Holm K, Kristiansson B *et al.* Different features of coeliac disease in two neighbouring countries. *Arch Dis Child* 1993;69:375–80.

Catassi C, Ratsch IM, Fabiani E *et al.* Coeliac disease in the year 2000: exploring the iceberg. *Lancet* 1994;343:200–3.

Logan RFA. Problems and pitfalls in epidemiological studies of coeliac disease. In: Auricchio S, Visakorpi JK, eds. *Common Food Intolerances 1: Epidemiology of Coeliac Disease.* Basel: Karger, 1992:14–24.

Mitt K, Uibo O. Low cereal intake in Estonian infants: the possible explanation for the low frequency of coeliac disease in Estonia. *Eur J Clin Nutr* 1998;52:85–8.

PATHOPHYSIOLOGY

Catassi C, Fabiani E, Ratsch IM *et al.* Is the sugar intestinal permeability test a reliable investigation for coeliac disease? *Gut* 1997;40:215–17.

Dieterich W, Ehnis T, Bauer M *et al.* Identification of tissue transglutaminase as the autoantigen of coeliac disease. *Nat Med* 1997;3:797–801.

Maiuri L, Auricchio S, Coletta S *et al.* Blockage of T-cell costimulation inhibits T-cell action in coeliac disease. *Gastroenterology* 1998;115:564–72.

Marsh MN. Gluten, major histocompatibility complex, and the small intestine. A molecular and immunobiologic approach to the spectrum of gluten sensitivity ('celiac sprue'). *Gastroenterology* 1992;102:330–54.

Nilsen EM, Jahnsen FL, Lundin KEA *et al.* Gluten induces an intestinal cytokine response strongly dominated by interferon gamma in patients with coeliac disease. *Gastroenterology* 1998;115:551–63.

Przemioslo RT, Lundin KEA, Sollid LM *et al.* Histological changes in small bowel mucosa induced by gliadin sensitive T lymphocytes can be blocked by anti-interferon γ antibody. *Gut* 1995;36:874–9.

Sollid LM, Thorsby E. HLA susceptibility genes in coeliac disease: genetic mapping and role in pathogenesis. *Gastroenterology* 1993;105:910–22.

CLINICAL MANIFESTATIONS

Catassi C, Fabiani E. The spectrum of coeliac disease in children. *Baillière's Clin Gastroenterol* 1997;11:485–507.

Collin P, Reunala T, Pukkala E *et al.* Coeliac disease – associated disorders and survival. *Gut* 1994;35:1215–18.

Corazza GR, Gasbarrini G. Coeliac disease in adults. *Baillière's Clin Gastroenterol* 1995;9:329–50.

Logan RFA, Tucker G, Rifkind EA *et al.* Changes in clinical features of coeliac disease in adults in Edinburgh and the Lothians 1960–79. *BMJ* 1983;286:95–7.

Page SR, Lloyd CA, Hill PG *et al.* The prevalence of coeliac disease in adult diabetes mellitus. *Q J Med* 1994;87:631–7.

Troncone R, Greco L, Auricchio S. Gluten sensitive enteropathy. *Pediatr Clin North Am* 1996;43:355–73.

DIAGNOSIS

Holmes GKT, Hill PG. Do we still need faecal fat? *BMJ* 1988;296:1552.

Sulkanen S, Halttunen T, Laurila K *et al.* Tissue transglutaminase autoantibody enzyme-linked immunosorbent assay in detecting celiac disease. *Gastroenterology* 1998;115:1322–8.

Swinson CM, Levi AJ. Is coeliac disease underdiagnosed? *BMJ* 1980;281:1258–60.

Volta U, Molinaro M, De Franceschi L *et al.* IgA anti-endomysial antibodies on human umbilical cord tissue for coeliac disease screening. Save both money and monkeys. *Dig Dis Sci* 1995;40:1902–5.

Walker-Smith JA, Guandalini S, Schmitz J *et al.* Revised criteria for the diagnosis of coeliac disease. Report of a working group. *Arch Dis Child* 1990;65:909–11.

COMPLICATIONS

Bai JC, Gonzalez D, Mautalen C *et al.* Long-term effect of gluten restriction on bone mineral density of patients with coeliac disease. *Aliment Pharmacol Ther* 1997;11:157–64.

Egan LJ, Walsh SV, Stevens FM *et al.* Coeliac-associated lymphoma. A single institution experience of 30 cases in the combination chemotherapy era. *J Clin Gastroenterol* 1995;21:123–9.

Holmes GKT. Mesenteric lymph node cavitation in coeliac disease. *Gut* 1986; 27:728–33.

Holmes GKT. Ulcerative jejunoileitis. In: Allan RN *et al.*, eds. *Inflammatory Bowel Diseases.* Edinburgh: Churchill Livingstone, 1997:431–5.

Holmes GKT. Neurological and psychiatric complications in coeliac disease. In: Gobbi G, Andermann F, Naccarato S, Banchini G, eds. *Epilepsy and Other Neurological Disorders in Coeliac Disease.* London: John Libbey, 1997:251–64.

Holmes GKT, Prior P, Lane MR *et al.* Malignancy in coeliac disease – effect of a gluten free diet. *Gut* 1989;30:333–8.

Howell WM, Leung ST, Jones DB *et al.* HLA-DRB, -DQA, and -DQB polymorphism in coeliac disease and enteropathy associated T-cell lymphoma. Common features and additional risk factors for malignancy. *Hum Immunol* 1995;43:29–37.

Lewis HM, Reunala TL, Garioch JJ *et al.* Protective effect of gluten-free diet against development of lymphoma in dermatitis herpetiformis. *Br J Dermatol* 1996; 135:363–7.

Sigurgeirsson B, Agnarsson BA, Lindelof B. Risk of lymphoma in patients with dermatitis herpetiformis. *BMJ* 1994; 308:13–15.

Swinson CM, Slavin G, Coles EC *et al.* Coeliac disease and malignancy. *Lancet* 1983;i:111–15.

Valdimarsson T, Lofman O, Toss G *et al.* Reversal of osteopenia with diet in adult coeliac disease. *Gut* 1996;38:322–7.

MANAGEMENT

Catassi C, Rossini M, Ratsch IM *et al.* Dose-dependent effects of protracted ingestion of small amounts of gliadin in coeliac disease children: a clinical and jejunal morphometric study. *Gut* 1993; 34:1515–19.

Janatuinen E, Pikkarainen PH, Kemppainen TA *et al.* A comparison of diets with and without oats in adult coeliac disease. *N Engl J Med* 1995;333:1033–7.

Kumar PJ, Walker-Smith JA, Milla P *et al.* The teenage coeliac: follow-up study of 102 patients. *Arch Dis Child* 1988;63:916–20.

Srinivasan U, Leonard N, Jones E *et al.* Absence of oats toxicity in adult coeliac disease. *BMJ* 1996;313:1300–1.

DERMATITIS HERPETIFORMIS

Fry L. Dermatitis herpetiformis. *Baillière's Clin Gastroenterol* 1995;9:371–93.

Garioch JJ, Lewis HM, Sargent SA *et al.* 25 years' experience of a gluten free diet in the treatment of dermatitis herpetiformis. *Br J Dermatol* 1994;131:541–5.

Reunala T, Collin P. Diseases associated with dermatitis herpetiformis. *Br J Dermatol* 1997;136:315–18.

Index

Also available

Asthma
by Stephen T Holgate and Romain A Pauwels

Benign Gynaecological Disease
by Eric J Thomas and John Rock

Benign Prostatic Hyperplasia (third edition)
by Roger S Kirby and John D McConnell

Bladder Cancer
by Michael Bailey and Michael Sarosdy

Breast Cancer
by Michael Baum and Harvey Schipper

Diabetes Mellitus
by Ian W Campbell and Harold Lebovitz

Diseases of the Testis
by Timothy J Christmas, Michael D Dinneen and Larry Lipshultz

Dyspepsia
by Michael J Lancaster Smith and Kenneth L Koch

Endometriosis
by Hossam Abdalla and Botros Rizk

Erectile Dysfunction (second edition)
by Roger Kirby, Simon Holmes and Culley Carson

Gynaecological Oncology
by J Richard Smith, Bruce A Barron and Andrew D Lawson

Osteoporosis (second edition)
by Juliet E Compston and Clifford J Rosen

Prostate Cancer (second edition)
by Roger S Kirby, Michael K Brawer and Louis J Denis

Respiratory Tract Infection
by Robert C Read and James E Pennington

Schizophrenia
by Shôn W Lewis and Robert W Buchanan

To order, please contact:

Health Press Limited
Elizabeth House, Queen Street,
Abingdon, Oxford OX14 3JR, UK
Tel: +44 (0)1235 523233
Fax: +44 (0)1235 523238
Email: post@healthpress.co.uk

Or visit our website:
www.healthpress.co.uk

Patient Pictures
Clinical drawings for your patients

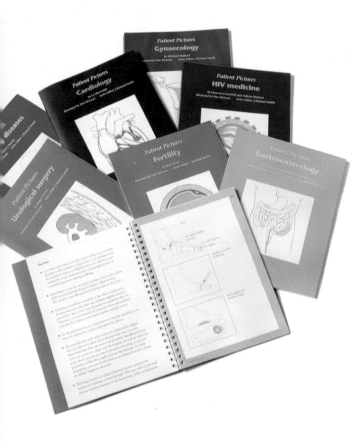

Bladder Disorders
by Eboo Versi and Timothy J Christma

Cardiology
by J Colin Forfar

Fertility
by Rod Irvine

Gastroenterology
by Penny Neild and Brian Gazzard

Genitourinary Medicine
by Simon E Barton and Antony Newe

Gynaecological Oncology
by Andy Nordin

Gynaecology (second edition)
by Michael Stafford

HIV Medicine
by Duncan Churchill and Valerie Kitch

Respiratory Diseases
by Peter J Barnes

Rheumatology (second edition*
by John D Isaacs

Urological Surgery
by Roger S Kirby

To order, please contact:

Health Press Limited
Elizabeth House, Queen Street,
Abingdon, Oxford OX14 3JR, UK
Tel: +44 (0)1235 523233
Fax: +44 (0)1235 523238
Email: post@healthpress.co.uk

Or visit our website:
www.healthpress.co.uk